THE GREATEST ENERGY ALWAYS PREVAILS

INTERESTING INSIGHTS INTO ADVANCED NATURAL MEDICINE

VOLUME 1

Amy,
I hope you enjoy this work
as much as I have. :)
Good Luck in School

THE GREATEST ENERGY ALWAYS PREVAILS

INTERESTING INSIGHTS INTO ADVANCED NATURAL MEDICINE

VOLUME 1

DR. HENELE E'ALE

PUBLISHING

ISBN: 978-1-61466-002-6

No Limit Publishing Group
123 E Baseline Road, D-108
Tempe AZ 85283
info@nolimitpublishinggroup.com

This book was printed in the United States of America

No Limit Publishing
No Limit Enterprises, LLC
1601 E 69th Street, Suite 200
Sioux Falls, SD 57108

Disclaimer

This volume contains opportunities to experience natural medicine and in doing so to gain a more robust understanding of the gifts that it has to offer you and your family. The suggestions at the end of each chapter are designed with the utmost safety for you in mind.

Still, this volume and subsequent volumes are designed to promote a healthy transformational process that gradually builds each week and as such may lead to some temporarily unpleasant experiences consistent with a natural healing process.

As such, it is possible that a particular suggestion offered may unintentionally conflict in some way with the directions of your existing physician. *In these cases we urge you to consult with your physician before attempting any activity or assignment that may potentially compromise the directions of your physician.*

Further, if you have reservations, doubts, or an unwillingness to participate in any suggestion we recommend that you refrain from it completely.

By participating in the suggested experiences within this volume you are agreeing to these terms and to taking full and complete responsibility for the outcome and for the most important gift you will ever earn… your health.

Namaste.

Acknowledgements

Aloha!

I come from a family of teachers. It is our collective profession.

As a devoted teacher, I can appreciate the desire to provide my students with every possible advantage aimed at their immediate development and future success. My job as a teacher is to place my students in a position to surpass me so that future generations can benefit. Ultimately, we are all stepping stones for future generations, and I take a great deal of pride in my participation in this process.

To that end, I welcome teachers to copy excerpts from this and future texts for classroom purposes without any fear of reprisal—provided that the excerpts are not full chapters and are not for sale.

I ask all teachers and students to respect the energy of this request, and I wish each of you good luck in your educational endeavors.

You are needed—perhaps now more than ever before.

Dr. Henele

Dedication

This text is dedicated first and foremost to my Father and Mother for their unwavering support. Thank you for believing in me when I failed to believe in myself. Thank you for teaching me to look for What's Good in all things.

This text and all that is good in me is dedicated to my incredibly awesome son, Sol Xavier Ealy. Thank you for being my inspiration to be a better Father. Thank you for helping me walk my talk. You are the light of the new house.

I also dedicate this text to members of my family—both living and living without their bodies. Thank you for investing so much love into me. I hope that I have made each of you very proud.

To my mentors—Dr. Theron Chapel, Dr. Vincent Medici (Professor S.), Dr. Mona Morstein, Dr. Walter Crinnion, Dr. Michio Sankey, Dr. DoAnn Kaneko, and the incomparable Ana Forrest—thank you for investing in me and trusting me with your healing wisdom.

To my students and my patients—thank you for teaching me how to be a better doctor in the truest sense of the word. Thank you for trusting me.

Finally, I dedicate *The Greatest Energy Always Prevails* to my love, Jessica. Thank you for being my light in the darkest of times. You have done more for me than you will ever realize, and for this, I stand devoted to you.

Dr. Henele a.k.a HL a.k.a Daddy a.k.a the Dude a.k.a Dr. H. a.k.a Your H.

Contents

Foreword By Dr. Nicole Gerard

My journey with Dr. Henele began in large part because of my emerging desire to study nutrition. For as long as I can remember, I watched as my mother struggled with a life-threatening illness. Thankfully, my mother was able to heal using natural therapies, and it was her Healing Process that inspired me to become a natural healer.

I remember my first nutrition course with Dr. Henele. Sitting in class, his knowledge and enthusiasm kept everyone engaged. I remember thinking, "I want to know what he knows!" There are special people in this world who have the true gift to teach, and Dr. H. is certainly one of them. I remember his passion for nutrition and his lectures regarding the body's innate ability to heal. Dr. Henele encouraged me to continue my journey at the Southwest College of Naturopathic Medicine and Health Sciences. Little did I know how much natural medicine was about to change my life!

Four years later, I began studying with Dr. Henele again as a medical student. He helped me feel increasingly confident in my abilities as a Naturopathic Doctor. I've seen him on an unending quest for knowledge and understanding. And what he learns he shares. Each time I study with him, he helps me solidify my knowledge more and more. Dr. Henele has taught me how to think like a healer. And it is a gift that is easy to appreciate.

I've watched him as he works with his patients. He listens to them, cheers them on, is encouraging, and is always in a truthful and genuine way. He taught me how to teach my patients, while also involving them in their own Healing Process. What he teaches in his classrooms mirrors how he teaches his patients. Dr. Henele teaches everyone to understand how amazingly resilient, yet delicate, their body truly is. He teaches you how to appreciate your body by caring for it naturally.

In helping him proofread this text, I now understand even more how deeply Dr. H. cares about healing. I enjoy reading what has taken him years of experience to acquire and develop. I admire his constant pursuit of functional research. I enjoy the connections he makes between Eastern and Western philosophies of healing. Dr. Henele has created an extraordinary text with a natural medicine perspective that teaches you how to listen to your body, interpret what it is saying, and respond by making good decisions that lead you into health.

Dr. H. embraces a dominant theme in his teachings— the cultivation of energy. He has convinced me that without sufficient energy the Healing Process cannot begin, but natural energy therapies can be incredibly effective. Dr. Henele has taken what is taught in naturopathic medical schools, and has elevated it to a higher level by teaching how intelligently the body is designed, and how to intelligently utilize the best of natural medicine. He consistently refers to your body's "Sophisticated Simplicity," while providing a strategy for selecting the appropriate natural therapies for the given situation. In this work, Dr. H. teaches so many things. I've never read anything that so clearly connects the body, the cell, and energy with the emotion of living.

I also enjoy how Dr. H. has a way of simplifying complicated concepts.

My favorite chapter of Volume 1 is definitely "The Art of Eating Healthy." Dr. H. explains what Eating Healthy really means. As I read the chapter, I couldn't help but revel in the amount of interesting information. I remember thinking, "I want to know what he knows." Now, thanks to his teachings, I believe that I do. Even better, I believe that I can really make a difference!

It is rare that a book comes along that clearly explains what Naturopathic Medicine is all about. *The Greatest Energy Always Prevails*, teaches. It informs. And above all, it encourages participation as you learn. Each chapter is a conversation that you will enjoy. In fact, each chapter offers you the opportunity to take that conversation to the next level by making simple changes your body can really feel.

As a student who has read many things medical, I smile saying, "I have not read a book like this."

If you have hungered for more knowledge, then I know in due time you'll be smiling too.

Nicole Gerard
Doctor of Naturopathic Medicine
Class of 2011

I Believe That Inside Each Of Us Lives A Healer

I believe that the wisdom of our healer within speaks with the intention of Love and from the universal collective consciousness, the Father we all share. Thus, our heart has the divine right to speak first and be heard as a guiding feeling, above all other thoughts.

I believe that life conditions us to silence our intuitive voice in favor of a rational mind that confuses our heart's wisdom with learned behaviors, second thoughts, and excessive analysis.

After all, what is, *is what is*. The Truth lives in how we feel. How we feel *is* how we feel no matter the second thoughts that attempt to rationalize away our heart's intuitive wisdom.

So what energetic purpose is served by placing our most precious emotions on internal trial, such that our own wisdom needs the justification of the rational mind?

For it is these very emotions, first spoken from the heart, that have the unique gift of leading us to our happiness, and of making our decisions in life obvious and simple.

After all, what could be more rational than leading with Love in all our endeavors?

Is there any other emotion that makes more sense?

What is more essential to happiness, joy, and satisfaction in life than Love?

I believe that within each of us lives the hope for a better future—for not only ourselves, but also for our families.

A future free from manipulative deceit, abuse, greed, and judgments.

A future that does not entertain fear or console apathy.

A future that feels the way our heart's wisdom describes life to us—filled with excitement, promise, and goodwill.

A future that we have created together—one that we can all participate in and be proud of.

For this vision to manifest itself, the time has come for us to listen to the healer within for guidance and ultimate delivery.

From many comes one so that many may come again.

One Love is Our Destiny.

One Love of Ourselves. One Love of Each Other. One Love of Our Home, Mother Earth.

The time has arrived for us to elevate our consciousness as one people to this pursuit.

Humanity's Greatest Energy is our collective ability, beating as One Heart, to embrace Love no matter the obstacle.

We are more than we have allowed ourselves to become, and yet our beauty remains living among millions of beating hearts and bright eyes.

I believe that together the healer within will elevate us to a collective beauty that we have only dared to dream about before.

I believe *The Greatest Energy Always Prevails.*

I believe Love is Our Greatest Energy.

I am honored to share with you sacred information passed down for generations that is highly effective and so dear to my heart.

I am grateful to you for your loving interest in yourself, in your family, and for your curiosity in natural healing.

Namaste. I salute the healer within you.

Dr. Henele

Welcome

We have a wonderful undertaking to accomplish together. For me, I have the opportunity to share with you interesting insights into the interrelationship between your health, your thoughts, your emotions, and the energy of your life from the perspective of your body, your organs, and their cells. My task is to present to you an incredible story about the unification of health in a way that inspires your appreciation for each unique aspect of life itself. When you think about your body, I want you to think, "WOW! That makes a lot of sense!" And then more importantly, I want you to be able to go and do something productive about it.

For you, the opportunity is to see your body and yourself from a revolutionary perspective that enhances what you already know, and that seeks to answer what you don't know. From personal experience, I know that life presents many questions that we have wanted answers to. Each chapter is dedicated to satisfying your curiosity for this exact purpose. For you, the opportunity is to see Advanced Natural Medicine for its gifts, and for its extraordinary relevance in today's *newer is always better, bigger is always better* imbalanced world. In essence, you have the opportunity to learn how to listen to your body so that you can make fantastic decisions on its behalf. I want you to feel incredibly confident in your ability to care for your body and, ultimately in doing so, how to care for yourself. How does that sound?

You will find that my writing style purposely violates a number of accepted standards in the field of writing, including my complete avoidance of maintaining proper tense and grammar. I have chosen this method of delivery to create a unique learning atmosphere whereby you and I can mimic the intimacy of a classroom and hopefully avoid the rigid boredom that health and large texts can sometimes be reduced to. My hope is that the writing style comes across as engaging, humorous, clear, participatory, easy to read, and that it allows for complete emotional involvement. I may say things that you strongly agree with, and I may say things that you strongly disagree with. My satisfaction is in knowing that you are passionately engaged with the topic, because that's when the best learning takes place.

The Greatest Energy Always Prevails is really one comprehensive text that I have decided to divide into three smaller volumes so that I would be able to get this healing information to you without delay. In Volume 1 of this book, the foundation is laid for a thought process that will help you maximize the effectiveness of advanced natural therapeutics. In Volume 2, we will apply this thought process to each individual system of the body, learning how the Cycle of Influencing Energy® affects each individual organ, its function, the energy it can produce, and how it can affect your energy fields and your emotional states. In Volume 3, we will unify Volumes 1 and 2 into a functional skill set for cleansing your body, calming your mind, and transforming any negative thought process or situation into a positive energetic outcome.

Along the way, each chapter has been organized to sequentially build on the previous chapter, while also engaging your sense of curiosity and adventure. Each chapter begins with a principle of healing followed by subchapters that are organized to support your understanding of the immediate chapter topics. Your time spent in each subchapter will be well worth it once you reach the chapter's end. At the end of each chapter, you will find two additional subchapters—"Listening to Your Body," and "What You Can Do to Cultivate Energy Today." It is in these last two subchapters that you will find activities designed to help you enhance your education through experiential learning. The strength of Advanced Natural Medicine is in the experience of positive energetic outcomes. In the final two subchapters of each chapter you will be presented with activities that will help you interpret what your body is saying to you, as well as invite you to explore relevant aspects of Advanced Natural Therapeutics.

Our mutual success in the pursuit of these goals will be realized as you develop the confidence to apply various skills for promoting health naturally. It is my intention and hope that the lessons you learn throughout this text will last you and your loved ones a lifetime. The development of what you are about to read is the result of fifteen years of dedicated study and practice. What you are about to read is a culmination of literally tens of thousands of years of human civilization's collective knowledge regarding healing. I know that the key to understanding Advanced Natural Medicine lies in the ability to thoughtfully apply relevant information. It has been an absolute joy of mine to learn this wisdom, update it for modern times with the help of recent scientific research, and develop the material in a way that I hope will be delivered in an encouraging and engaging way.

Your body is beautiful, asks for so little, and gives so much in return. It is a wonderful study in efficiency, conservation, sustainability, and energy production.

I hope that I can enthusiastically convey my understanding of our most precious gift—the body in which we live every day.

Dr. Henele
Doctor of Naturopathic Medicine

CHAPTER 1: FATIGUE

The #1 Root Cause of All Disease

Interesting Insights to look for in this chapter:

- Fatigue is your body's first warning sign of impending disease.
- Fatigue sets the stage for the Bio-accumulation of infections and environmental pollution.
- Stress is more to your body than just an emotional reaction.
- Naturopathic Doctors do it without harm.

Principle of Advanced Natural Medicine #1:

Where there is space, there is movement.

Where there is movement, there is energy.

Where there is energy, disease cannot exist.

The Root Cause of All Disease is Fatigue

Where there's space, there's movement; where there's movement, there's energy; and where there's energy, disease cannot exist. This is a principle that I teach to help my students understand that the body has and needs space within it. More often than not, space in the body is filled with water. In fact, the healthy adult body can range anywhere from 65 percent to 75 percent water. Where there's adequate space, there is space for the exchange of nutrients, there is space for the exchange of cellular waste, and there is space that's going to facilitate the movement of the fluids within the body. As a result of space and movement, the potential for energy to be created becomes an efficient reality. An energy that promotes health—an energy that makes everything go. Thus, this phrase becomes our first foundational thought process from which every future principle is based on. In order to heal, we *must* first have the energy to heal. Without energy, natural healing does not work. Without energy, the body will not heal. No other consideration even closely rivals this concept. Its truth is simple and plain.

This establishes the concept that the root cause of all disease is fatigue. When we look into any pathology book (and of course these are thick textbooks, often with more than two thousand pages, filled with centuries upon centuries of information), we see that fatigue is always a primary component of the symptom presentation for any pathology. Pneumonoultramicroscopicsilicovolcanokoniosis—the longest word in the English language—is actually a Lung disease. Guess what symptom occurs with it? Yes indeed—fatigue. With fatigue—a primary component of every disease process—it becomes a unifying principle in the study of health. I think this fact is too often dismissed, which is perhaps why we have been taught so little about our amazing body. Imagine if every child was taught how to eat, play, rest, and think to maximize energy production—what a Louis Armstrong wonderful world it would be.

For example, we're told over and over again that inflammation is bad. But a Naturopathic Physician is going to question this because inflammation is actually a sign that the body has initiated a healing response. Have you ever been told that inflammation is essential healthy tissue regeneration and repair? Have you ever been taught that energy is essential to these processes taking place?

You see, it doesn't matter what part of the body or organ system is affected. It doesn't matter if it's a Lung pathology or a disease of the Large Intestine. It doesn't matter if it's a disease of the Stomach, a disease of the Liver, or a disease of the Nervous System—it all comes back to the same thing. Fatigue—a lack of energy. The disease process began because the body didn't have enough energy to keep that area clean, to keep the cells in that area healthy, and to keep the Immune System strong and on alert. *A fatigued body is a body ripe for infection.*

So what we are saying, "If that's the case, what happens if we look at this idea of health from an energy or energetic perspective?" What happens if we look at it and say, "If I give the body everything that it needs to produce energy, what might be the outcome then?" What happens when we practice from this perspective is that a person may have eight, nine, ten different health issues going on. What if we respond without getting overwhelmed and simplify the problem? What if we say, "You know what? That's a lot going on, for certain. I'm going to give you everything your body needs to produce energy to clear up the picture." Then something amazing happens—six, seven, eight of those things have the potential to fall off the board within weeks. What we're left with is the true picture of what's really going on—the underlying contributing factors to disease. With a clear picture, medical decision-making improves by leaps and bounds.

Make sense so far? Well let's continue on then.

Who's Responsible for Your Health?

One of the things we've been led to believe in our culture is that our health is not our responsibility. When we get sick, we have been taught to believe that it's not our fault, and that it happens to everyone. We're led to believe that no matter what we were doing, no matter how good a person takes care of themselves, that disease is inevitable. This self-defeating thought process is a BIG problem, and one that we will work together to overcome throughout this text.

Imagine that you could take the greatest care of yourself, that you could *eat healthy* in a way that we will define together. Imagine that you could play (exercise), and keep your stress levels low. Imagine that you are in full control of your health, and that you are able to confidently navigate the storms that life presents to you. What a wonderful world we could create if we completely accepted responsibility for our own health. Of course, navigation requires tools and skill. A little touch of good luck never hurt either.

Previously, you may have entertained the notion that if you get sick that it's not your fault. It's not your responsibility. That your health is not your responsibility. And what does this set the stage for in your life? Let me guess. It sets a stage for you feeling like it doesn't matter if you're educated about your body, how it works, and how to care for it or not. Let me get this straight, you and your body are in this thing called life together and YOU don't matter?! What a preposterous idea! Are you someone who knows more about your job than your body? Doesn't that stop to make you think? How can you do your job without knowing how to do your job? How can you take care of your body without knowing how to take care of your body?

We've been given this amazing, incredible gift of life in a human body, and yet too many of us have little or no concept of how to care for it. Let me offer this additional thought: To know more about how to download something from the Internet than you know about where your Liver is or how it functions, sets you up to make bad health decisions. To know more about balancing your bank accounts than balancing your pH or other essential nutrients for self-maintenance is to invite fatigue into your life, leaving you susceptible to inevitable disaster.

One of the proposals that I'm making is this: If you know more about your body, than you ultimately know more about how to take care of it. And in knowing more about how to take care of it, the foundation is going to be set for the production of energy. If all you know about your body is how it works to produce energy and what you can do to facilitate that, then you know 98.827329 percent more than most people currently know out there. Yet this is what we need to change—agreed?

Understand this about education, decision-making, and saving money. The more you know about your health and how easy it is to maintain, the better your decision-making will become. The better your decisions regarding your health, the more money you will save, the more energy you will produce, and the better you will feel. Knowledge of your body's needs keeps you AWAY from the doctor's office. Knowledge keeps you away from the operating table. Knowledge keeps you away from having to rely on twelve to fifteen medications, which unfortunately, is becoming more and more a reality for our senior population.

As a quick aside, when you talk with most seniors, they're on at least five medications. Many of them are on ten or more medications. With each new medication, the side-effect profiles become more prominent until they avalanche. Can we really call it living when the day is dictated by a pill schedule and the outcome is fatigue—often replacing one symptom for two new ones? Understand that the body was not designed to be able to handle that amount of daily chemical load in the first place.

So then let's begin right here, right now with healing. Do you believe that you have the power to improve your health? Hopefully your answer to each one of these questions was "yes." Let's keep moving forward. Do you believe that your health is within your control? Hopefully your answer to each one of these questions was "yes." Let's keep moving forward. Are you ready to learn how to produce energy? Hopefully your answer to each one of these questions was "yes." Let's keep moving forward. Who is responsible for your health? The person in the mirror. Good. Then let's keep moving forward.

The Powers That Be

Practicing preventative medicine is practicing medicine focused on energy production, first and foremost. The powers that be (and they are really, really big) want us to believe that our health is not in our control and that our genetics are erosive and degenerative. Without hope of healing, diagnoses—especially for serious diseases—can be quite daunting. Choosing to heal and believing that it can happen is something that I think as a culture we have to wrap our minds around and say, "I can do this. If I know more about how to produce energy, then I believe I can prevent—in the truest sense of the word—disease." Can this indeed be a reality that energy production is the key to overcoming disease? The answer is yes, absolutely. I'm living proof of it.

Why Haven't We Taken Fatigue More Seriously?

There are a couple things at work here. Number one is we've been led to believe that we're just getting old, when the reality is that we're not getting enough. We're not getting enough nutrients, we're not getting enough playtime, we're not getting enough sleep, enough laughter, enough sex, enough touch, enough sunshine, enough enjoyment, enough satisfaction, enough peace, enough love in our lives. We're not getting enough life, and unfortunately, that's what getting old is for too many of us.

Fatigued, we learn to cope with not getting enough by swinging the pendulum in the opposite direction as we attempt to correct these deficiencies by getting too much. You see, when the body is deficient in energy, our body transforms from an energy producing, detoxifying powerhouse into what is known as a *Bio-accumulating Organism.* Without energy, we Bio-accumulate too many pesticides, too many chemicals, too much work, too much sitting on our butts, too much aggravation, too much insomnia. We Bio-accumulate too much stress, including taking in the stress from those around us. *When the amount of stress in our bodies and in our lives exceeds our ability to produce energy, disease is the only possible outcome.* The first warning sign of the impending doom, known as disease, is fatigue. In this way, being tired all the time, and not having enough energy to enjoy life is the canary in the coal mine. My question to you is, have you been listening to what your body is telling you when you are fatigued?

As mentioned earlier, we've also been misled to believe that there's nothing we can do about the way we feel, which is a flat-out lie. It's a lie that's been told to us by corporate marketing from a multitude of industries that want our hard-earned money. They sell us the idea that degeneration is a fact of life, and that a little pill will take care of the problem. If that pill doesn't work, or it causes something else, no problem—there's a second pill for the side effects. This cycle goes on and on and on, and twelve pills later, it starts dawning on us that something doesn't feel right. That maybe there is a better way. After trust is exhausted, brave people walk into a Naturopathic Doctor's office thinking, "I can't afford to deal with any negative impressions I may have had about you people and the witchcraft voodoo, hokey, shaman thing that's been keeping me from coming in." Patients come in and realize we're just normal people with good medicine, good education, and a strong desire to help. It usually comes out like, "Wait a minute, you're just a normal doctor." And we reply, "Well, yeah." And they go, "Oh, cool." And we go, "Yeah."

The third factor in this whole soap opera of taking fatigue seriously is that we've been miseducated. Not only are we undereducated about our amazing body, but we're miseducated. In many cases, this misinformation leads us to completely misinterpret what our bodies are attempting to say. For example, did you know that in order for the Immune System to launch into action against a foreign invader the body often has to feel it? That's right. Without pain as a signal that something is wrong, the Immune System has little to no direction as what to do. Pain is the body speaking plainly that something is wrong, and it often is an essential part of the Healing Process. But we'll expound on this in later chapters.

It is simple things like this that have been mistaught. Our bodies are always talking to us, because life is a mutually beneficial relationship. We have needs. Our body has needs. And when both sets of needs are fulfilled, life is awesome and grand. And yet something keeps getting lost in translation, because we're only choosing to hear what the TV or Internet is telling us. There is a very real education problem when a person's understanding of their amazing body is limited to what can be conveyed by thirty-second advertising spots. This is the intention of this text. Read it thirty seconds at a time if you need to, but get the whole thing done so that you can learn the language of your body.

I believe that everyone takes their health seriously, but I also believe that people have not been drinking from the same fountain of knowledge. I also cannot deny that unfortunately, many people don't take their health seriously enough until it becomes a problem for them—until it becomes disease. Listen, one of the worst thought processes to indulge in is, "Oh, I'm just tired, I'll get over it. I'll push through this wall." Then two, three years later—as that fatigue has continued on—you have a real problem that will cost more financially and emotionally to correct.

That's why I am teaching you to listen to the early alarm. It makes very little rational sense to wait for fatigue to turn into disease. Certainly, there are different types of fatigue such as physical, emotional, and mental fatigue. Can you differentiate between them? Absolutely. But to your body, there is no difference—fatigue is fatigue regardless of the cause. The impact on the body is the same. This is the beauty of the body. The body is about Sophisticated Simplicity.

Your body can't differentiate between the effects of fatigue from physical stress or emotional stress or mental stress because the body says, "We're all in this together, to heal, I treat all of them the same. I need nutrients, rest, movement, and change in lifestyle. Give me these things, and I will give you energy for health."

The thing to remember, and it is *that* important, is that a lack of energy leads to the body becoming a Bio-accumulating Organism due to suppressed immune function. This is a nice way of saying your body becomes a trash bin. As the dominoes begin to fall, suppressed immunity leads the body to accumulate pollution. The pollution that we are constantly exposed to, that our bodies normally get rid of very quickly, now builds up in the tissues, and alters the physiological functioning. With the Immune System offline, the stage is set for infections to start taking hold in the body because all the microorganism germs are trying to live, too. And what better to live on than a susceptible, Bio-accumulating, weak host?

If you're a microorganism germ, who would you rather attack—somebody with a suppressed Immune System or somebody with a strong Immune System? You're going to take the person who's fatigued, who has a weak Immune System, because you're going to be able to feed off of them until they figure out how to get rid of you.

If this is sounding like someone you know, give a nod.

Quick Recap and Toxic Relationships

Tired? Check. Bio-accumulating pollution? Check. Suppressed immunity? Check. Infections? Check. Well, without energy there's even more to the story, believe it or not. Fatigued, your body will Bio-accumulate common cellular wastes as well as other people's emotional garbage. That's right—when you are tired, you are more likely to take on other people's toxic energy and have difficulty getting rid of your own. You might be thinking, "Doc, you're crazy." This may very well be true, but think about your life for a moment. Ever had a child or a spouse, a colleague, a relative, or a friend who consistently took you for granted? Guess when? When you were fatigued, and perhaps you thought the best thing to do was to ignore your body's needs for the needs of someone who was entirely capable of taking care of themselves. Ever cleaned up behind a messy teenager or had to stay late at work because a coworker didn't finish their work? Now you're getting it. When do these moments occur? When you are already fatigued.

These are the relationships that are toxic to us when people—who we often call our friends—are just taking and taking from us, or just dumping all their problems and not reciprocating and listening to ours. And guess whose fault that is? Look in the mirror. ☺ To not give credence to emotion as a real and ever-present aspect of a person's health, and/or a contributing factor to fatigue is, tragically ignorant. Because we've all experienced the effects of destructive emotions in more depth than many of us would care to admit.

Why Haven't We Taken Fatigue More Seriously? Continued...

Now, back to the body. Depending on which systems are genetically weak or simply overrun from pollution exposure or infection, this is where the *cellular adaptation theory* —what we call disease—takes place that we'll talk about later. For now, let's go one step further. You're fatigued, you've become a Bio-accumulator, and your Immune System is offline. This we now understand. At this point, depending on where your genetic weaknesses are in the genome, you will start to experience disease first. It's not rocket science. I actually have a degree in Mechanical Engineering. I studied rocket science, and it's really hard. Health is not very difficult to understand, but it does take an understanding of the logic of your body and how it all works together to be able to understand the simplicity of it.

We also do not take fatigue seriously enough due to our use of stimulants. Our culture is addicted to stimulants to compensate for the experience of fatigue. Coffee, energy drinks, sodas, refined sugar, and recreational drugs are our attempt at self-medicating, and they ultimately do more harm than good. There is a better way. We are always going to rely on what we know. Whether it's an MD who knows pharmaceuticals, a Naturopathic Physician who knows herbs and nutrients, or a patient who knows information that a friend of theirs discovered on the Internet. We're going to do what we know. And what we know is that when the motor is sluggish, we need a stimulant to get our act in gear.

I think we do the best we can with what we know how to do. Am I selling something? Of course I'm selling something—I'm selling the idea of energy, the feeling of health, and I'm selling a plan on how to get there. I know this plan works because it's worked for me and thousands of people like me. It has worked repeatedly because it's not based on greed, but rather on how your body is designed to work. Let me encourage you for a moment. It is time to learn about your body and how to take care of it. There's no bad time to learn how to care for yourself. Right now is the perfect time and you CAN do it.

My job is to help you set the stage for success. I know that the more you understand your body, the more you will come to appreciate the need for energy and take fatigue with the level of seriousness it demands—because now you will know what to do about it and why. My job is to educate, and your job is to participate. This is all we can ever ask of each other, and I think it's a very fair deal.

Why Do We Get Sick? Why Do We Get Diseased?

We next talk about why people get sick, because that's always the big question. Well, why did this happen? I've had patients in front of me with cancer, serious digestive disorders, asthma, and much worse. They all want to know the same thing: "Why did this happen?" And there's such resignation for them to say, "Well, this is the luck of the draw. My number got called, and I'm the person who got cancer."

Nothing happens in our bodies by accident. Our bodies are incredible. When you think about it—at any moment in time, there are literally more than four billion biochemical reactions occurring simultaneously, and without error. We're able to go to sleep, wake up, go through our day, and then go back to sleep again and all seemingly without having to have conscious control over our body. But yet, things just accidentally happen? Yeah, right.

I think that's a point of view that's hopeless and something that is marketed to us to accept. It doesn't matter what you do, it doesn't matter how much you know, it doesn't matter how well you take care of yourself—at some point, you're going to get sick, it's going to be very serious, and we're going to have a pill for it, or we're going to have a surgical procedure for it. Really? Is that what we have to look forward to as we age? Why can't we look forward to feeling great each decade? Why can't we look forward to understanding what our bodies need each and every decade and provide for it? Of course, we're going to get sick from time to time. That's how it works, and that's how our Immune System stays sharp. But that doesn't mean that we have to get diseased. After all, there is a significant difference between getting sick and getting diseased.

Getting sick is the body's ability to encounter environmental pollution or a microorganism germ, and then having energy available for the Immune System to respond to it expertly to get rid of it. That's a sign of healing—getting sick. It's why a little sniffle every now and then is actually productive—it's training the Immune System how to remain efficient.

While getting sick is natural, getting diseased is a problem. We don't actually *get disease.* Disease is something that develops in the body, typically following extended periods of fatigue. To date, this has taken place because of the lack of education we have discussed previously, and the excessive amounts of stress we have asked our bodies to endure. We are, without a doubt, one of the most undereducated cultures when it comes to our own bodies.

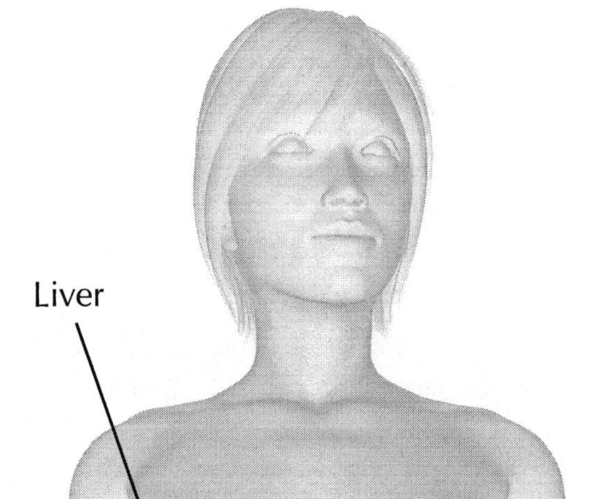

Figure 1.1
Notice how the majority of the Liver is on right side. *Live Right.*

A good example of this is considering how many people know something as simple as where their Liver is? Take your right hand. Hold it up high. And now gently pat the lower portion of your right Rib Cage. Hear that dull thud? Congratulations! You just found your Liver. Your Liver is on your right side. Here's an easy way to remember it: Live Right. (See **Figure 1.1**)

Something as simple as knowing where your organs are is paramount for you to know how to take better care of yourself. If we were to go one step further and understand what the Liver does, then now we're really playing with power. I believe that the vast majority of us are ready to be proactive about our health once we know how wonderful a clean and well-cared-for body feels. When I teach health and healing from the body's perspective, this amazing feeling in the classroom develops that most people can't get enough of—I hope you're already feeling the same way.

When we look at disease, we want to understand what causes fatigue. Typically, we don't have to look much further than the following:

- Nutritional Deficiencies
- Delayed Food Allergies
- Dietary and Environmental Pollution
- Infections
- Scar Tissue
- Negative Internal Dialogue

These are the biggest players for virtually everyone, and I would assume that they would cover at least 95 percent of the underlying causes for fatigue. Certainly, most cases of fatigue can be traced to combinations of these six factors. If we add to these factors a lack of satisfaction in our lives—along with emotional stress that comes from fear, frustration, guilt, isolation, feelings of inadequacy, and all the things that erode our sense of self—then what we have is an incredible combination of stressors for the body to endure. The foods that we eat, how we feel, the things we breathe in, and the deficiencies in our diet all set the stage for fatigue, and ultimately, Bio-accumulation of pollution. Once our body is in Bio-accumulation mode, we become a breeding ground for microorganism germs to proliferate in our bodies. What a perfect food we become for the bad bugs!

When combinations of these factors begin to overwhelm the body, the experience of fatigue becomes cyclical. We seek stimulants like refined sugar, coffee, and energy drinks because we are fatigued, but these all help feed the infections, while shutting down the Immune System at the same time. As infections and pollution accumulate, our ability to produce energy becomes greatly compromised. At some point, we have to learn how to break this self-defeating cycle.

Exposure vs. Susceptibility

Now, one of the things that we have to explore when it comes to explaining why people develop disease is the concept of exposure versus susceptibility. In our society, we're led to believe that if somebody has a bad bug, we're going to get it. If you're in your office sitting in your cubicle and somebody in the cube next to yours starts sniffling and sneezing, we automatically think: "Oh no, oh no, I'm going to get that!" Well, you know what? That is miseducation hard at work.

What Advanced Natural Medicine teaches us is that whether or not our bodies express disease is the result of a combination of exposure AND susceptibility. It's not enough for a person to just be exposed to something. A person also has to be susceptible to the germ. If your Immune System is low because you are fatigued, that makes you susceptible. If your diet is nutritionally deficient, if you are fatigued because of long hours at a thankless job, if you have become a Bio-accumulator, if you are eating foods that your Immune System is attacking, then the likelihood that your body will express disease goes WAY up because you are more susceptible.

However, when you're exposed to something and your Immune System is healthy, when you're energetic and you're feeling good, the likelihood is that you may feel a symptom or two, but it'll be very brief. In many cases, you may not feel anything because, guess what? That microorganism germ that came into your body, found its worst nightmare. The worst nightmare for a germ isn't a vaccine. *The worst nightmare for a germ is a healthy Immune System.* Your immune cells are constantly on the prowl to devour any germ, and anything that's not supposed to be inside you. When the Immune System is healthy and it has the energy to do what it needs to do, a germ comes into your body and it runs for cover—it runs screaming away.

When your Immune System is weak, when it's been suppressed, when it doesn't have what it needs to support itself—in other words, the health of your whole body—something happens. Germs get into the body, and they start setting up residence. They start to take over the tissues, and they begin to produce symptoms of illness. And if that goes on for long enough, that can turn into disease. What was a little sickness can turn into a disease when a body is fatigued and susceptible.

The key ingredient to understand is that it's not just exposure that determines whether a person gets sick or develops disease. It is exposure and susceptibility. Susceptibility is determined by how much stress you have in your life, and how much energy you have the ability to produce.

When the amount of stress that a person has in their life—from all factors—exceeds the ability to produce energy, disease is the only outcome that can happen. I can't stress this enough—*when the amount of stress that a person has in their life exceeds the ability to produce energy, then disease can be the only outcome.* That's where we take it back to the first thought process of natural healing: there's space, there's movement; where there's movement, there's energy; and where there's energy, disease cannot exist. In order for disease to become a reality, a person must be susceptible. In order for a person to be susceptible, they first must be tired. That's what that statement is all about.

Emotion and Energy Production

We've established that it's only in a low energy state that we can get sick. That's what we haven't been taught well enough until now. It's only in a low energy state that we can get sick, because the Immune System can't do its job.

Part of what sets us up for high energy or low energy is the relative sense of satisfaction within our lives. People who are satisfied with their lives, and who are feeling good about the direction of their lives, have a tendency to produce energy more efficiently, have stronger Immune Systems, and make better decisions. It's amazing how people who are happy with the direction of their lives and who are following their dreams are typically in a much better state of health. It's an energy that the body produces that Chinese Medicine and Ayurvedic Medicine understand. Interestingly enough, Western Biochemistry understands this energy too.

It's this energy that runs through us, animates us, and is responsible for so many things going right—second after second, day after day, year after year—within the body.

It is interesting to me that one thing we all understand in every single culture, is how we feel. We have developed entire languages based on this premise of trying to communicate and express what we are feeling inside to others. We understand emotion because it is one of the things that, from the time we are born to the time we pass away, we experience every day.

Emotion and health are not independent realities. Emotional contentment is an indication of the health of a person. People who are happy and satisfied are in a better state of health than people who are not. I think we've all had that experience of at least some satisfaction in our life, perhaps most easily understood when in love with someone else. Ever heard someone say that they are sick and tired of being in love?

Exactly, it doesn't sound right because it's probably never been said before. Love is potent medicine—it heals, it reduces stress, and it helps us keep everything in perspective. Love is resilient, and something we will discuss in detail and in a very real way at the end of this book. The main point to understand is that certain emotions help cultivate energy, while others speed its consumption.

When Are Pharmaceuticals Part of the Answer, and When Are They Part of the Problem?

One of the things that I think we have to impart is an understanding about when pharmaceuticals are part of the answer, and when they become part of the problem. We need to explore an understanding of when Advanced Natural Medicine provides a better solution than pharmaceuticals.

Certainly pharmaceuticals are the answer in emergent situations, and there has never been a medicine better suited for emergent situations than the one we now employ. Pharmaceuticals in emergent situations have the ability to take a person—who in other times would have died from infection or a systemic shut down of their body's vital organs, and keep them alive. When dealing with emergency situations, there isn't a medicine on par with current Western conventional medicine.

However, this medicine is not as effective as I believe medicine should be when dealing with chronic situations. I'm not talking about emergent situations. I'm talking about chronic situations where a person's lifestyle and experiences have obviously brought them into a state of ill health and disease. My question for you is this: Can you name a pharmaceutical medication that produces energy as a side effect? I've looked for one for years, but haven't been able to find one.

Chronic ill health, a disease state that involves fatigue, begs for change—lifestyle change. That's what the strength of Advanced Natural Medicine offers patients. It is offering a plan of wholesale, multilevel lifestyle changes that a patient can participate in throughout twenty-eight-day cycles of healing, because that's really—for whatever reason—how the body heals. The body heals in twenty-eight-day cycles. Maybe it has something to do with the cycles of the Moon and our body being two-thirds to three-quarters water… I don't know. But what I do know is that if a participant is making productive lifestyle changes on multiple levels, that person's energy will continue to build and build and build. This occurs because in Advanced Natural Medicine we're able to do something, I think, that is not of this world—we're able to identify obstacles to cure and help the patient remove them from their life.

Maybe the obstacle to cure is a germ that's in the body for months and months, causing infection. Well, let's find it, determine precisely how to kill it, and let's get it out of the body. Maybe the obstacle to cure is that your diet is not supporting your specific needs for energy production. Either you're eating food that your Immune System is attacking due to delayed food allergies, or you're not getting enough nutrients in your diet. Well, great, let's get that obstacle to cure out of the way too. Maybe you've been exposed to too many environmental chemical pollutants. Perhaps you've lived in too many brand-new homes, worked in too many sick buildings, worked in too many toxic environments, and your body's accumulated too much pollution. Well, let's clean your cells, get that stuff out of your body, and let's remove that obstacle to cure as well.

When we approach the return to health like this, something amazing happens. When we remove the obstacles to cure and set you up for success, your energy increases every twenty-eight days for as long as you are disciplined, follow the plan, and continue with your lifestyle changes. And because your energy increases, your Immune System gets stronger. As your

Immune System gets stronger, you get stronger. As you get stronger, your Energetics improve, and guess what? Something magical happens that we'll learn about in chapter two—your moods improve. How you interact improves. How you communicate improves. If you are dealing with a chronic degenerative condition, then the key is identifying the obstacles to cure and acting on them intelligently. Advanced Natural Medicine affords you this opportunity.

It's not uncommon for me to encounter a patient who comes into my office with ten or more medications. In fact, I've had patients with as many as twenty-two different medications that they were taking on a daily basis. Talking pharmaceuticals, twenty-two medications simultaneously is not okay. We have very limited research on the effects of drug-to-drug interaction and how this might exponentially increase the side effect profiles of both medications. And that's for only two medications. We have even less research on how three medications interact, and we have almost none—and if we do have research, I've never seen it—of four or more pharmaceutical medications and how they interact. Yet every day, millions of Americans are taking more than four pharmaceutical medications simultaneously. Combine that with daily stress, excessive sugar consumption, and the chemicals in our food, and what you begin to reveal are some likely suspects for why someone develops disease.

The thing that Americans don't know is that conventional medicine by definition is called allopathic medicine. If we go to *Taber's Medical Dictionary*, we read that the definition of allopathic medicine is: "The art of cure founded upon differences, by which one morbid state is removed by inducing a different one." By definition, what they are saying is, "We are going to try to cure you by replacing a symptom for a new symptom." Huh?

With the use of *morbid* state as a term, marketing pharmaceutical medications to the public would be virtually impossible. Pharmaceutical companies wouldn't be able to sell their medications if they said, "Hey, we're going to take away your morbid condition by giving you a morbid condition." Nobody would go for that medicine. So what marketing conveniently did was change the term "morbid condition" to "side effects." Because side effects are conditions that everybody can accept. People rationalize all of this by saying, "Well, you know, that's just the consequence of getting sick, and now this is something that I'm going to do to get myself better." Side effects—They're easier to sell.

Guess what the new terminology is for morbid conditions? Alternative adverse events. Word play and marketing at its best. Attack your competition... Alternative Medicine... covertly. Absolutely brilliant in a very diabolical kind of way, don't you think?

So if pharmaceutical medications have side effects, then do natural medicines like nutrients and botanical medicines have side effects? Yes, most natural medicines promote the production of energy. If somebody wants to accuse me of helping someone produce more energy and getting their Immune System healthy, then accuse me right away. That's the side effect of the medicine that I practice. In all fairness, are there some toxic herbs and some nutrients that are toxic at high doses? Yes. Are these herbs and high doses often needed? Fortunately, no.

It's knowing when and how to use these medicines that makes Advanced Natural Medicine so special. So what we're doing is making the case for pharmaceuticals in emergent situations. You want to stay healthy, you want to restore health in your body, you want to overcome chronic illness by increasing energy production? Natural medicine—it makes sense. Moving forward, this is how the two medicines can work together—by knowing which situation is appropriate for their application.

Final thought. One of the things that we have to understand is that a doctor can only provide what they're taught. A Medical Doctor (MD), conventional, medical, Allopathic Physician, is taught pharmaceuticals. A Naturopathic Doctor (ND) is taught clinical nutrition, botanical medicines, pharmaceuticals, and much more. We are all taught how to diagnose, we are all taught basically how to think, and then we're taught how to treat. An Allopathic Physician, an MD, is going to treat using pharmaceuticals. An ND is hopefully going to treat from a much broader selection of therapies. This is because we are taught a larger selection of natural therapeutics designed to stimulate sustained energy production, that will overcome the effects of fatigue.

What Natural Medicine Brings to the Table

As Naturopathic Physicians, we are going to study pharmaceuticals, but we're also going to study Clinical Nutrition and Botanical Medicine, and natural therapeutics like Homeopathy, Massage Therapy, and Spinal Manipulation. We're going to study Acupuncture and Traditional Chinese Medicine, Yoga, and principles of Ayurvedic Medicine. We're going to study all the therapeutic approaches that people have been using successfully for more than five thousand years. This is what's amazingly awesome about Naturopathic Doctors. We have an incredible number of tools that are just waiting to help people. All we're really asking for is the opportunity. Let us show you what we can do.

What natural medicine brings to the table is a bridge to a new lifestyle, predicated and founded upon the cultivation of energy. What natural medicine does at its strength is say, "I understand that your body, in order to heal, has to engage the *Vis Medicatrix Naturae*—the vital force that lives within us. I understand that the most physical representation of that vital force that we know today is present within each cell and what Biochemistry and Physiology have figured out as organelles called Mitochondria and their production of a substance called ATP, adenosine triphosphate."

If we, as physicians, can remove the obstacles to cure, the things that are blocking the production of ATP… If we, as physicians, can also give you the things that we know your body needs to produce ATP, then the vital force—the *Vis Medicatrix Naturae*—is engaged. When it's engaged, your body is so incredibly intelligent that it starts to heal on its own. It does what it's designed to do. I promise you that your body is designed to heal. Your body is also designed to maintain homeostatic balance. Imagine attempting to perform any of these tasks essential for living without energy. *Energy is the essential cofactor for healing and homeostatic balance.*

For example, let's say at some point you cut yourself. Of course the cut healed. You didn't have to think about it, you didn't have to tell your body what to do, your body did it instinctively. But the real question is this: How often do you take your amazing body for granted?

What happens as we age is that we say to ourselves, "Well, when I was younger I used to heal real fast, now I don't heal as well." Well, part of that might be a little drop-off in genetic reproduction. But maybe a bigger part of that—and the reason why the genome is less efficient—is that we haven't been nourishing it for a couple of decades. We haven't learned to become caretakers of our most precious gift. We've been exposing our body to too much pollution, too much stress, too much neglect. And thus we feel old and tired. Coincidence?

Maybe the reason why our bodies don't respond as we would like in our thirties, forties, fifties, and beyond, is because we in our undereducation, haven't known how to take care of them. That's what the following chapters are designed to remedy.

The intention of this text is to teach everyone about how emotion—something we all understand—unifies the body and provides an excellent tool for assessment. You are going to understand how an emotion both reveals how an organ is being affected and how emotion affects an organ. You are going to learn how an organ functions, and what changes take place because of that. As a result, what does that mean to your production of energy? What does that mean to your body's pH? What other things start to suffer because of the problems we've created? We're going to start with emotion, but you're soon going to understand that your body doesn't care whether emotional reactions are causing the fatigue, or whether nutritional deficiencies, fatigue, direct injury, or trauma are causing the fatigue. Your body doesn't care. Your body doesn't care if it's environmental pollution or infection that's creating the obstacle to cure.

Your body doesn't care, because your body is responsible for keeping you alive. It has to treat damage from various stressors exactly the same—it attempts to heal from them.

The Definition of Natural Medicine

Naturopathic Physicians are primary healthcare practitioners just like their conventional colleagues. The difference that we want to establish is between the MD, the allopathic Medical Doctor ,and the ND, the Naturopathic Doctor. Our ability to diagnose is very similar. How we get to the understanding of what the diagnosis is, and the assessments necessary to discover it also is similar. Maybe we look at it from a broader perspective that accounts for diet and emotion—factors that are often dismissed. Our thought process for deciding on treatment is different. But ultimately, a diagnosis is a diagnosis—it's either right or wrong. Gastritis is Gastritis. Insomnia is Insomnia. Brain Fog is Brain Fog.

The big difference is in our basic definition, which then helps us develop treatment plans. Allopathic medicine is, by definition from *Taber's Medical Dictionary*, "the art of curing founded on differences, by which one morbid state is removed by inducing a different one." This is currently marketed today as "side effects" or "alternative adverse events," as we mentioned earlier. By definition, Naturopathic Medicine is, "the art of curing founded upon utilizing the body's innate natural healing forces. In doing so, Naturopathic Medicine acts to assist the body's natural restoration of energy production and balanced homeostatic function." So, by definition, we are very different. Our collective goal to help the people we serve is very noble and unified, but our approach, in most cases, is often quite different.

Naturopathic Code of Ethics

When we study the foundation of Naturopathic Medicine, we learn that it is founded upon six healing principles. The Naturopathic Doctor holds these Codes very dear.

THE FIRST PRINCIPLE IS THE HEALING POWER OF NATURE

We believe that nature provides everything we need to restore energy production and homeostatic balance. And how do we know it works? Because we can *feel* it. Healing is one of the most commonly shared human experiences. Healing occurs over and over again, and the Naturopathic Doctor is very proud to work in harmony with nature, rather than trying to control it.

THE SECOND PRINCIPLE IS TO IDENTIFY AND TREAT THE ROOT CAUSES

What we are constantly in pursuit of are the root causes of disease identified as obstacles to cure. What is getting in the way of your body working optimally? We believe that the body doesn't make many mistakes—that the body is designed to work for decades. The only time that we encounter problems are when our body encounters obstacles that hinder it. The Naturopathic Doctor's job is to find the root causes of disease, such as fatigue, and help you remove them from your life.

THE THIRD PRINCIPLE IS TO DO NO HARM

In an effort to help someone, we can't afford to induce a morbid state. We are not going to attempt to make someone better by giving them something that could make them worse. This is where we have a fundamental difference with conventional allopathic medicine, and that's okay. It's okay for us to have a difference of opinion because we're not in an emergency room. We're not treating emergent conditions, we're treating chronic conditions, acute conditions, and conditions that can be prevented. That's our strength. They have to have a perspective of, "We might have to give you something that might cause some other harm just so we can keep this other organ alive while we're saving your life." So give them that. One morbid condition for another is okay in the right circumstance. One morbid condition for another loses its effectiveness when treating chronic conditions.

THE FOURTH PRINCIPLE IS THE DOCTOR AS TEACHER

Doctor comes from the Latin word *Docere*, which means to teach. The job of the Naturopathic Physician is to educate and empower you. So as you're going through your Healing Process, you learn how to make us obsolete. My greatest pleasure in life is when a patient doesn't need me anymore because we've restored them to health. For a Naturopathic Doctor, that's what we live for, what we are passionate about, and what keeps us coming back for more. Wonderful is the opportunity to share with someone this brilliant medicine that can have a positive influence—not only on a patient's life, but also on the lives of their family members.

THE FIFTH PRINCIPLE IS TO TREAT THE WHOLE PERSON

We look at the person from an encompassing, holistic perspective—a concept called the Cycle Influencing Energy that we will discuss in chapter two. You are made up of so much wonder, that we want to make sure you have the opportunity to appreciate how you fit together. What's nice about our journey is that we've stripped away the minutia, and we have kept the interesting substance. Together we are going to develop an easy-to-apply thought process that I hope will serve you a healthy lifetime.

THE SIXTH PRINCIPLE IS THAT WE PRACTICE, PREACH, AND LIVE PREVENTION

It is said that an ounce of prevention is worth a pound of cure. People who know how to care for their bodies are likely to care for them in a productive way. I also like the old adage: Pay me now, or pay me later... but you will pay me.

LISTENING TO YOUR AMAZING BODY

How does your body tell you that it is fatigued and that the stage for disease has been set? Read from the questions below and candidly answer Yes or No.

1. Are you currently dealing with a chronic disease or illness?

   Yes No

2. Are you currently taking more than two pharmaceutical medicines?

   Yes No

3. Does it take you more than fifteen minutes to get out of bed in the morning?

   Yes No

4. Do you regularly feel sleepy at work after lunch or when you are driving home?

   Yes No

5. Are you easily annoyed or frustrated?

   Yes No

6. Do you look forward to or wish you could just stay home?

   Yes No

7. Do you get sick all the time?

   Yes No

8. Do you exercise less than thirty minutes two times per week?

   Yes No

9. Do you drink multiple cups of coffee, sodas, or energy drinks each day?

   Yes No

10. Do you feel tired, exhausted, or frequently overwhelmed?

   Yes No

If you answered "yes" to one of these questions, then you are fatigued and likely have become a Bio-accumulating Organism. While each question is a good indicator of fatigue, questions 5. and 6. in particular can be early warning signs of fatigue.

What You Can Do To Cultivate Energy Today

One of the ways that we can begin to cultivate energy is by becoming aware of where we are losing energy, and then making small changes in our lifestyle. To better assist this exploration, answer the questions below and then let's make one simple resolution for improving the space within your body.

1. What stresses you out? Write exactly what comes to mind immediately. Don't judge yourself, just write.

____

____

____

____

____

____

____

____

2. How long did it take you to write down your first answer to the question above?

____

3. What have you done recently for yourself that brings you happiness?

____

____

____

____

____

____

____

____

____

____

____

4. How long did it take you to write down your first answer to the question above?

____

Questions 1. and 2. help identify where you lose energy, and to what extent your thoughts are preoccupied with that loss of energy. For example, if your list of things that stresses you out is lengthy, obvious, and took little time to uncover, then there is a strong likelihood that you are losing energy due to these stressful events. Questions 3. and 4. are meant to identify where you gain energy, and to what extent your thoughts are preoccupied with the pursuit of your own happiness.

If you were faster in answering question 3. than you were in answering question 1. this is very good. It means that you spend more time looking for what is good, and for what brings you happiness. The ability to look for what is good is an excellent skill to possess. It means that you think about happiness more than you allow stress to affect you. If you also wrote more answers for question 3. than question 1. this is also very good. It confirms that you have more positive thoughts than negative ones. It means that it is easier for you to discover what makes you happy.

If you were able to answer question 1. faster than question 3. and in more depth, you are probably spending too much time with negative thoughts and situations. Ultimately, these stressors are leading to damage within your body, and are contributing to fatigue.

CREATING A HEALING JOURNAL

Throughout this text, you will be presented with the opportunity to participate in the experience of natural medicine. One of the opportunities in front of you will be to create a Healing Journal so that you can record your experiences, as well as the personal growth that is to come. Begin a Healing Journal by using either a traditional diary, electronic diary, Internet blog, or audio or video recording to document your experiences while you journey through this text. The process will be a whole lot of fun.

RESOLUTION #1

Select one of the following experiences that you will treat yourself to this week so that you can begin developing the skill of finding What's Good in your life as you simultaneously create more space in your body for movement and energy. Take a picture of your face before and after the experience, and post both pictures on your refrigerator or bathroom mirror as a reminder of how good creating space can feel.

1. Sixty-minute professional or student massage.
2. Sixty-minute Yoga class, Pilates class, or Cardio class.
3. Sailing, Surfing, Flying, Hiking, or Cycling excursion.
4. Preparing a meal that is one hundred percent Organic/Free Range.

HEALING JOURNAL RECORDING

Record in your Healing Journal your moods, thoughts, and positive experiences with this resolution. Also record in your Healing Journal a little bit about what you are hoping to learn and/or experience while you work through this text.

Good Luck!

CHAPTER 2: CYCLE OF INFLUENCING ENERGY®

The Thought Process of the Advanced Natural Healer

Interesting Insights to look for in this chapter:

- Your body is designed to heal using Sophisticated Simplicity.
- Love feels the same in every country, in every body, every day, for all time.
- The body offers multiple points of entry for natural therapeutics to cultivate energy.
- Positive Internal Dialogue is the essential key for successful healing.

Principle of Advanced Natural Medicine #2:

Your body is designed to heal.
Sophisticated Simplicity makes it all possible.

Stress is Stress is Stress

Your body does not differentiate between various types of stress. Stress from internalized emotion causes as much cellular damage as stress from an acidic diet. The body responds to all stressors in a similar fashion by drawing on its energy resources to initiate a proactive healing response that involves your Immune System.

Translation: *Your body is designed to heal.* And because it's designed to heal, it needs to perform with Sophisticated Simplicity. Sophisticated Simplicity is a concept that can be summed up in this way: While the action of healing may be somewhat complicated, the logic that the actions are based upon are quite simple. Understanding Sophisticated Simplicity is a way of appreciating all that goes into a Healing Process without necessarily needing to know everything that goes into it. The logic of Sophisticated Simplicity treats cellular damage from all stresses exactly the same way. Your body cannot function efficiently with a thought process that goes something like this: "I'm going to treat stressful damage caused by excessive Scar Tissue differently than stressful damage caused by Fast-foods or sodas." To respond differently to different stressors would invariably lead to complication, and the subsequent inefficiencies that would result from that.

Your body's ability to perform with Sophisticated Simplicity is, in fact, its greatest attribute. Here's why: All your body cares about is damage, not what caused it. What I want you to understand is that all stress causes damage at the cellular level. All the body cares about is repairing damage, because your body is responsible for the continuance of life. Once damage occurs from stress, a signal is sent throughout the Nervous System, a pain signal. *The pain signal is the beacon for the Immune System and all of your body's resources to go into advanced healing mode.* Your body doesn't care if the stress is due to hurt feelings, or due to lack of money to pay the rent. Your body doesn't care whether the stress is from a tragedy, a trauma, or just a nutrient-deficient fast-food diet. Your body doesn't care. Stress is stress is stress, and damage is damage is damage—regardless of where it's coming from. The key concept to understand is this: Stress from any source causes cellular damage. The similar response to damage—regardless of cause—is your body's first Sophisticated Simplicity.

What's interesting is that your body has a definitive and logical process for regulating its performance, day in and day out, for many decades. To best understand how your body 'thinks' using the principle of Sophisticated Simplicity, I present to you the Cycle of Influencing Energy®.

The Cycle of Influencing Energy® (CoIE)

The Cycle of Influencing Energy® (CoIE) is a paradigm for advanced natural healers that is designed to integrate multiple aspects of your body's various perspectives into one unifying concept. Simply put, this is my way of sharing with you what your body is saying so that you can understand its language and make great decisions for your health.

You see, your body is always talking to you, and it's always telling you what's going on, what it needs, and how far you can push it before it needs a rest. All your body is asking you to do is listen and utilize awareness to participate in this mutually beneficial relationship.

CoIE: Emotion – Our Common Language

The Cycle of Influencing Energy® looks at your body from the following integrated perspectives: 1) Anatomy—how your body is structured, 2) Physiology—how your body functions, 3)Biochemistry—how your body produces energy, 4) Energetics—how your body distributes energy, and 5) Emotion—how you feel as a cumulative result of aspects 1 through 4. (See **Figure 2.1** on next page) To best begin our journey into understanding the way the body thinks, we will begin our discussion with something we all know very well—emotion.

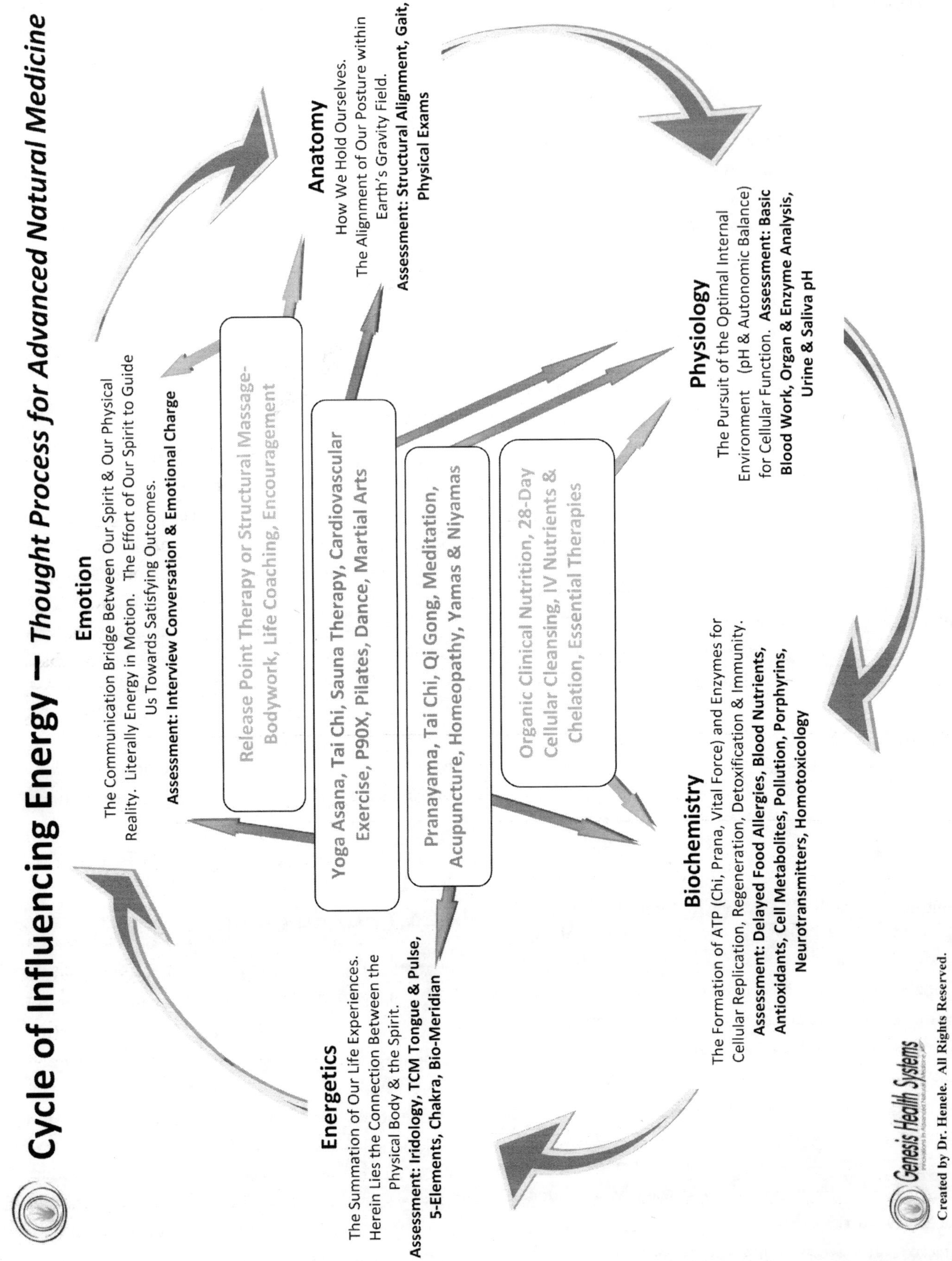
Cycle of Influencing Energy – Thought Process for Advanced Natural Medicine
Emotion
The Communication Bridge Between Our Spirit & Our Physical Reality. Literally Energy in Motion. The Effort of Our Spirit to Guide Us Towards Satisfying Outcomes.
Assessment: Interview Conversation & Emotional Charge
Anatomy
How We Hold Ourselves.
The Alignment of Our Posture within Earth's Gravity Field.
Assessment: Structural Alignment, Gait, Physical Exams
Physiology
The Pursuit of the Optimal Internal Environment (pH & Autonomic Balance) for Cellular Function. Assessment: Basic Blood Work, Organ & Enzyme Analysis, Urine & Saliva pH
Biochemistry
The Formation of ATP (Chi, Prana, Vital Force) and Enzymes for Cellular Replication, Regeneration, Detoxification & Immunity.
Assessment: Delayed Food Allergies, Blood Nutrients, Antioxidants, Cell Metabolites, Pollution, Porphyrins, Neurotransmitters, Homotoxicology
Energetics
The Summation of Our Life Experiences. Herein Lies the Connection Between the Physical Body & the Spirit.
Assessment: Iridology, TCM Tongue & Pulse, 5-Elements, Chakra, Bio-Meridian
Release Point Therapy or Structural Massage-Bodywork, Life Coaching, Encouragement
Yoga Asana, Tai Chi, Sauna Therapy, Cardiovascular Exercise, P90X, Pilates, Dance, Martial Arts
Pranayama, Tai Chi, Qi Gong, Meditation, Acupuncture, Homeopathy, Yamas & Niyamas
Organic Clinical Nutrition, 28-Day Cellular Cleansing, IV Nutrients & Chelation, Essential Therapies
Genesis Health Systems
Created by Dr. Henele. All Rights Reserved.

Figure 2.1

Emotion is the common language that we all share. A person who is frustrated in America—regardless of what they're frustrated about—often feels that frustration internally. It is emotion that generates physical, visceral, gut-level reactions throughout the body's systems. That same exact experience—regardless of what causes the frustration—is what another person feels in England, France, Zimbabwe, Australia, China, Antarctica, or on the Moon. It doesn't matter where it is experienced, or by whom—the human body is pre-wired to respond to emotion similarly so that it can continue to perform in spite of any adversity.

We all feel emotion the same way. It has been said that math is the universal language. Well I would argue that emotion is the universal language of life. Emotion unifies us in a way that many of us have not necessarily acknowledged. Regardless of language, cultural upbringing, gender, religion, or age, sadness feels the same way to each person. Frustration feels the same way to each person. Anger feels like anger. Fear feels like fear. In fact, all the energy draining emotions feel the same way to every person in the world, and your body is designed to react pretty much the same way. If an emotion causes cellular damage, then your body will attempt to heal using the principle of Sophisticated Simplicity.

On the flip side—and what's really awesome about how emotion unifies us—is that energy cultivating emotions work within your body's Sophisticated Simplicity as well. Calm feels like calm. Enthusiasm feels like enthusiasm. Confidence feels like confidence. It feels good to report to you that a person who is in love in America feels love and experiences it just like a person in Mexico feels and experiences love. If we can understand—as we will go into more depth later—which emotions drain energy, which emotions cultivate energy, and how we have the freedom of choice to engage either side, then we accept an awesome power and responsibility. Working with and from conscious emotion, we can fully promote our own healing. Working from a place of consciousness affords us a freedom that is too seldom realized.

Thankfully, I've learned something through my life experiences that is an inescapable, undeniable truth. A truth that I am glad to share with you because it's something you already know. Love energy is the most powerful energy we've ever known, and probably will ever know. Love energy heals everything. Love energy wins out over it all. Love is the greatest energy, and as such, it will always prevail. Love energy affords the Mitochondria of our cells to most efficiently produce energy in the form of ATP.

Emotion is an amazing communication bridge between our spirit and our physical reality. Something is going on within life that is far greater than just this, us, or our body. We have a tendency to think of ourselves in terms of our bodies, and we identify ourselves with our bodies all the time. This is great and wonderful, because for now, we live in our bodies. But we're also something beyond that. I think anyone who's had a near-death experience, or who believes in life after death and things of that nature, the question—at least in my mind—is always, "Well, what do we take with us?" The only thing I've ever been able to come up with during meditation that's made any sense, is that we take with us how we feel. How we feel is our experience, our truth. How we feel is a summation of the states of health of our physical body, and how we perceive life around us. The product of this summation is our emotional state. The cleaner our body, the clearer our mind will be; the clearer our mind, the easier it will be to hear the desires of our spirit.

I'm sure this has been said before, but emotion is e-motion—energy in motion. Tell me one decision in your life, one event, one instance that has been completely devoid of emotion. I've asked this question of thousands of people, and no one has been able to come up with an answer—because even the absence of emotion evokes an emotion. The purpose of emotion is awesome. Emotion is how our spirit communicates into this physical reality to enable us to make decisions. Our emotional state is our guide. What's important to understand is that to make the clearest decisions, we need a clean body so that any impairment in health does not cloud our decision-making. It is no accident that we base the large majority of our decision-making on things that make us feel good. We do this because feeling good is a very attractive force that we seek to re-create again and again. When things don't make us feel good, that is a wonderful opportunity to learn and change our decision-making. Problems ensue when we place ourselves in negative cycles of redundancy with our decision-making. The result often is that we are quick to find what we don't like, yet we spend too little time pursuing what turns us on. You see, we've been given this great assessment tool for life called a human body, and the better we care for it, the easier and clearer our decision-making becomes. *Like something, repeat it. Don't like something, listen to your body and Change It. Life is kind of that simple.*

Hopefully, as we grow and learn to listen to ourselves more, our emotions will guide us toward more satisfaction. In doing this, we begin to create a wonderful opportunity to be shining lights for each other. Perhaps a friend looks at you and says, "You know what? You're always happy. I'd like to be that way, what did you do?" And you reply, "Well, I just started being myself." To which they say, "Hmmm. That looks like it feels good. I'm going to start doing that, too." This can be your reality when you listen to your body as your guide.

Something amazing happens with emotion, for better or for worse. There are two types of emotions—energy cultivating and energy draining. So you can get an idea of how it works, let's consider the energy draining emotion of sadness.

As it stands, emotion in the Cycle of Influencing Energy® is at the pinnacle for a reason. Emotion leads because it's something we are all masters of experiencing, if not yet masters of working within. Looking at **Figure 2.1** again, emotion influences our Anatomy, which is our physical body, and how we hold ourselves within the gravity of Mother Earth. When someone around us is sad, it's often not hard to see the dejected face and slumping shoulders. This is emotion influencing Anatomy. Anatomy is something we know a little bit about, but we're more familiar with how we feel. What most of us don't know is that how we hold our body affects how the structures underneath the Skin perform, our Physiology. If we are out of alignment from slumping shoulders, and we are working hard just to hold the body upright, then our breathing will become shallow and oxygen will be deficient throughout the body. As oxygen becomes relatively scarce, the Heart compensates by pumping faster to take more blood with less oxygen to the cells, because the cells still need the amount of oxygen they need for the Mitochondria to produce energy. It only stands to reason.

Next up is Biochemistry, how the cells produce energy. If the Physiology is off due to sadness, then the cell's ability to produce energy will be compromised due to the lack of oxygen needed to produce energy. With cellular energy deficient, the cell's predesigned functions—including detoxification, will slow noticeably. From an energy standpoint, the Lungs also become compromised due to lack of movement. As a result, the stage is set for infection in that tissue. Ironically, one of the energy draining emotions associated with the Lungs is sadness. So this energy draining Cycle of Influencing Energy® will only act to further embed the sadness, or grief, into the body.

In essence, sadness often leads to slumping shoulders. Slumping shoulders keeps the Lungs from taking in the amount of oxygen necessary for cellular energy production. Deficient oxygen leads to a deficit of energy, otherwise known as fatigue. And fatigue leads to a deficiency of energy moving through the energy channels of the body, which ultimately manifests as grief.

So what's the key to healing from an energy draining cycle like this? Using your consciousness to Change It. Change the habits that are reinforcing an energy draining cycle into an energy cultivating cycle, which is a topic covered in every chapter of this book.

This is the power of emotion. Emotion can heal us, or it can contribute to our demise. It can operate as an assessment tool and report to us what our body is feeling, and it can change how our body performs on a physical and energetic level. Ultimately, our emotions are a common language. They are the easiest place to begin an in-depth understanding of health and the body's thought process for Sophisticated Simplicity.

Everything Is Connected— How Could It Be Any Other Way?

Is the study of Anatomy more than just how we hold ourselves in the field of gravity? Of course it is. But do we need to know every little nuance in order to understand our body's thought process? Absolutely not. Remember the understanding I want to convey to you is Sophisticated Simplicity. In future books I will provide much more functional information concerning Anatomy, and I will teach you how to read your body's history. But for now, simple is the key in all aspects.

As we turn our attention from emotion and Anatomy to Physiology, it's important to simplify the material. Our interest in Physiology—how the body functions—is in the following two aspects: 1) the autonomic Nervous System, which is how your body has been pre-wired to automatically control all functions, and 2) your pH, which is the alkaline-acid environment your body is designed to work within. *At a cellular level, the majority of cells prefer to live in a slightly alkaline pH environment because alkalinity promotes the highest production of energy.* Conversely, cells that are exposed to a regularly acidic environment consistently encounter damage because acid by definition breaks things down, and is therefore stressful to your body. As such, cellular energy production suffers, and the energy that is produced is often used for cellular repair rather than optimal cellular functioning. Think of alkaline pH as the body's optimal environment for energy production, and as a way for your body to conserve its own energy. Which is hopefully leading you to wonder how do I make my body more alkaline? That's a good question…

So your emotional state influences your anatomical structure, which influences your physiologic functioning, which then influences your biochemical production of energy. This is how your body works in an integrated approach for self-maintenance. So you can see how a feeling can cause real changes in your physical body. In fact, what you think and feel gets all the way down into the nitty gritty—the biochemical cell level.

Cells feel what you feel. How could it be any other way? Let me say that again, the cells of your body feel what you feel. You are not separate from your body—that's preposterous and a residual linear thought process proposed by René Descartes in the early 1600s that still infects world thought to this very day. It is an outmoded notion that works best with respect to math and Cartesian coordinates, but not with respect to the multivariable universe of your body. And guess what breaks down that linear thought process upon which so much conventional medical thought is based? Emotion. Which is why so many Allopathic Physicians have discounted its effects—it does not fit their model of the body. For their model of the body to be effective, the body must be isolated into independent units that seldom interact, and when they do, only interact in strictly controlled patterns. Your body is beautiful and amazing nothing is independent of anything else, least of all you from your body. Thus, a cell will always feel exactly what you feel because your cells are you and part of the whole team.

A cell's job above any other is to produce energy in the form of ATP (adenosine triphosphate). This is a beautiful thing. Talk to a biochemist, they're going to say, "Oh, yeah, ATP. I know about ATP." You talk to a Naturopath, you're going to say, "Hey, what's up with that ATP?" They're going to say, "Oh, yeah, I know about ATP. We also call that the *Vis Medicatrix Naturae*, the vital force." And you say, "Oh, cool. Okay, you got another name for it." Then you go to the Far East, and you visit China, Japan, or Okinawa, and what happens? You start talking about ATP. And they say, "Oh, okay, yeah. I've studied some Western medicine, I know about ATP, yeah. You know what we call that? We call that *Chi*." And you go, "Oh, that's pretty cool." Then you go to India, and you talk to some Ayurvedic doctors there. You say: "Hey, what about ATP?" And they say, "Yeah, we know about ATP. We call it *Prana*."

So many different names, but at the end of the day, all the good stuff looks and feels the same. When you are investigating your body according to the four hundred-year-old Cartesian linear thought process, consider that it really hasn't worked with respect to longevity. You also might want to ponder the possibilities of a cyclic, multivariable thought process based on Sophisticated Simplicity. At the end of the day, life is all about energy production, and what's so fascinating is that the Cycle of Influencing Energy® offers so many ways to cultivate energy. You can create energy from your emotions and thought, by how you decide to hold your body, or from how you breathe to create alkaline pH, or by nourishing your body with nutrient-dense Organic foods. *Every aspect of the Cycle of Influencing Energy® provides you with yet another entry point to cultivate energy in your body and your life.*

What's also interesting is that the Cycle of Influencing Energy® provides a way to understand degenerative disease processes. That is to say that the CoIE is neither positive nor negative. Rather, it's how you choose to work with or against yours and your body's needs that ultimately determines whether the cycles you create are cultivating energy or draining energy. That's right, produce energy or lose energy—it's all up to you. It's all within your control, and it has always been this way.

Progressing from emotional states to anatomical structures to physiologic functioning to biochemical energy production, at last we arrive at Energetics. Energetics is the study of how energy flows through the body, and the associations that are created throughout the body from the flow of energy. Energetics allows us to say that a particular emotion affects an organ, or that an organ is associated with a particular tissue. It's what allows you to understand that sadness affects your Lungs, and that the health of your Liver is associated with the health of your Tendons and Ligaments. I can almost hear the indignant skeptic asking: "But where is your proof?" To which I would respond, "Where is your proof that these associations do not exist? Seems to me that the Taoists and Ayurvedics have been expertly using these principles for more than five thousand years on literally hundreds of millions, if not billions, of people. That's either wisdom, or one mighty long and far-reaching scam."

Advanced Natural Medicine is for people who believe, and my job is to help explain things in easy terms. But even I don't suspect I'll be able to convince everyone. The funny thing about life is that everyone always tends to be right when it comes to believing what they want to believe anyway.

So with that aside, back to Energetics. Let's take a sneak peak at **Figure 2.2** and start with the Fire Element to illustrate some of the significance of this particular energetic. The Fire Element is said to include both the Heart and the Small Intestine. You have probably heard of Acupuncture, and know that the body has key locations where needles are placed to stimulate mystical energy pathways called *meridians*. Well, this is true. Your body has energy pathways that originate from the actual organ and travel up to the surface of the Skin to help distribute energy throughout your body. What's so beautiful about the practice of Energetics is that there is little difference between the organ and the meridian that flows from it. Thus, for the Fire Element the two companion symbiotic organs are the Heart and the Small Intestine. Why? Why do most hands have five fingers? That's just the way you're made!

Referring to **Figure 2.2** and continuing on with the Fire Element, some energy draining emotional states include Love Pain, a Sense of Unworthiness, Resistance to Change, Difficultly Accepting Defeat, Blame, Judgment, Feelings of Victimization, and Negative Internal Dialogue. This means that any of these emotional states leads to a disruption of Mitochondrial Energy Production and a loss of energy that results in fatigue, and ultimately, disease. The Fire Element also includes energy cultivating emotions like Courage, Acceptance of Change, Feelings of Encouragement, a Sense of Accountability, Positive Internal Dialogue, Satisfaction, Joy, Authenticity, and Love. This means that these emotional states lead to more efficient energy production in the Mitochondria—a condition that promotes more beneficial effects for you through the CoIE.

This is the power of positive thoughts, words, and deeds—they build energy. Of course, there are nutrients and botanical medicines that support the Fire Element. If that's not nifty enough for you then consider this: The health of the heart can be seen in the tongue, and heard in the voice. When you sweat during cardiovascular exercise, you are actually clearing stagnant Heart energy. The health of your Heart can also be seen by examining your blood vessels. Energetics teaches us that the Heart is most active in summer, and also most active between 11 A.M. and 1 P.M. Here are a few more interesting tidbits using Energetics… As the temperature rises, the Heart can become more energized. Red is a good color to stimulate Heart energy (as with a rose). Bitter flavors stimulate Heart energy, and also aid in enzyme production. How neat is that? To have a way to decode your body so that you are better able to listen to your body's needs. Sophisticated Simplicity.

Are Energetics For Real… Really, Real?

Let me give you a personal example of this. In 1999, I was on death's door. I had a love of my life—who was also my best friend—come into my apartment and tell me that she wasn't in love with me anymore. I was crushed, and something crazy happened to my body, that I still remember and say, "Wow, what a night!"

When she told me this, I fell down on the ground in tears, and my body went into convulsions. Now, you might think, "Oh, you were being dramatic. You were acting." Nope. This really happened. How my body reacted is how deeply I felt what was happening. I felt my heart break—physically break. What I know now is that this was a twisting and constriction of the Pericardial tissue surrounding my Heart. In that moment, something that began as an emotion quickly became physical and physiological, and I fell to the ground.

My body's systems started to shut down because of this. What was I feeling during this? Was I feeling sad? No. Was I feeling frustrated or angry? No. Was I feeling remorseful? No. What I felt was the same thing we all feel when our Hearts are broken—I felt pain. Pain is an incredible signal that damage has occurred. Was this event stressful? Yes. Damage was occurring throughout my entire body all at once, resulting in the collapse to the floor, the contraction of my body, and the convulsions. It was systemic, and it was all created by several words: "I don't love you anymore."

I can still feel those words to this day.

That night—after hours of lying awake in shock—I somehow went to sleep. The next morning, I woke up and saw something I had never even heard of before or since. In the toenail of each of my big toes was an obvious diagonal crack from the corner to the base. It was huge. It was bilateral. It was scary. I'd never seen anything like that. It was like somebody—while I was sleeping—came and tried to rip my toenails in half. It was obvious and visible. I only wish I had taken a picture.

After a few minutes of freaking out, I went into the bathroom mirror and saw a ghost. I had huge dark circles under my eyes. My Skin—which normally is quite radiant (I don't mean to brag)—was pale and pasty. My cheeks looked like they were falling off my face. I had lost three clumps of hair. I had three bald spots on my head where clumps of hair had fallen out. I also had a streak of gray running through my hair.

For anyone who thinks I'm sensationalizing this, I assure you that I am not. I looked in that mirror, and I saw a person who had aged, by fifteen or twenty years overnight—and not very well. I saw a person in front of me who was dying rapidly, that's how severe that experience was for me. What was the emotion?

Figure 2.2

Genesis Energetics - 5 Element Perspective

	Fire	Earth	Gold	Water	Wood	Accessory Fire
Yin Organs	Heart	Spleen-Pancreas	Lungs	Kidneys	Liver	Pericardium[1]
Yang Organs	Small Intestine	Stomach	Large Intestine	Urinary Bladder	Gall Bladder	Triple Heater-HPAxis[2]
Gland	Thymus	Pancreas	Thyroid, Parathyroid	Adrenals, Reproductive	Liver, Reproductive	HPAxis
Energy Draining Reactions				**Acidity - Sympathetic 'Fight or Flight' Dominance**		
Primary Root Cause	Love Pain					
Secondary Reactions (Coping Mechanism)	Unworthy of Joy, Love or Happiness	Excessive Concentration, Being Busy as an Escape	Grief (Extended Sadness)	Lack of Trust	Anger, Indecisiveness, Emotional Instability	Alone, Isolated, Neglected
3rd Level Reactions (Behavior Adaptation)	Resistant to Change, Acceptance of Defeat	Mental Chatter, Easily Overwhelmed	Keeping It Locked Inside, Unable to 'Let Go'	Fear of Unknown, Worry, Anxiety	Frustration, Impatience, Complaining, Timidness	Guilt, Excessive Thought
4th Level Reactions (Destructive to Self)	**Blaming Others, Hypercontrolling &/or Victimized Persona**					
5th Level Reactions (Destructive to Self & Others)	**Negative Internal Dialogue, Irrational, Vindictive &/or Judgmental Persona**					
Energy Cultivating Responses				**Alkalinity - Parasympathetic 'Rest & Digest' Balance**		
Healing Decision	**Courage, Belief, Taking Action for Positive Change**					
Primary Healing Skills	**Encouraging, Positive Internal Dialogue, Accountability, Appreciation**					
Primary Healing Responses	Loving, Satisfied, Joyful, Enthusiastic, Authentic	Rational Decision Making, Clear & Calm Mind	Forgiving, Truthful, Encouraging, Postive Communication	Trusting in Life's Perfection, Faithful, Belief	Patient, Peaceful, Confident	Investing In Family, Friends, & Passions Creating Community
Primary Nutrients	**Mitochondrial Energy Producing Nutrients, Chlorophyll & Organic Foods**					
Supportive Nutrients	Vitamin B12, Folic Acid, Vitamin E, Co-Q-10, Magnesium, Taurine, L-Carnitine, Essential Fatty Acids, Amino Acids	Vitamin C, Vitamin K, Calcium, Essential Fatty Acids, Digestive Enzymes, Amino Acids	Vitamin A, Vitamin D, Vitamin E, Vitamin K, Zinc, Probiotics, N-acetyl Cysteine, L-Glutamine , Glutathione	Clean Water, Vitamin C, Vitamin D, Vitamin K, Biotin, Calcium, Magnesium, Potassium, Sodium	Vitamin A, Vitamin C, Vitamin K, Alpha-Lipoic Acid, Taurine, Lecithin, Essential Fatty Acids, Glutathione, Amino Acids	Minerals, Amino Acids, Vitamin D
Botanical Medicines	Hawthorn Berry, Rosemary, Ginkgo Biloba	Peppermint, Spearmint, Ginger, Gentian, Rose Hips	Cordyceps, Licorice Root, Maitake, Astragalus Root, Lauracidin	Siberian Ginseng, Ashwagandha, Schisandra Berry, Nettles	Green Tea, Milk Thistle, Burdock Root, Turmeric, Reishi	Skull Cap, Passion Flower, Kava Kava, Gotu Kola
Associated Facial Features	Tongue	Lips	Nose	Ears	Eyes (Sclera)	Eyes (Iris)
Additional Associations	Voice	Smooth Muscle	Immune System	Reproductive Organs*	Uterus	Body Temperature
Associated Fluids	Sweat	Saliva	Lymph	Urine & Semen	Tears	Cerebral Spinal Fluid
Tissues	Blood Vessels	Skeletal Muscle	Skin, Sinuses, Lymphatics	Bones	Fascia & Sinews**	Dura Mater - Endocrine
Most Active Seasons	Summer	Late Summer	Autumn	Winter	Spring	Early Summer
Most Active Times	H 11a-1p, SI 1p-3p	Sp-P 9a-11a, St 7a-9a	L 3a-5a, LI 5a-7a	K 5p-7p, UB 3p-5p	L 1a-3a, GB 11p-1a	P 7p-9p, TH 9p-11p
Imbalance Climates	Heat	Dampness	Dryness	Cold	Wind	
Energy Directions	South	Center	West	North	East	
Energy Colors	Red	Yellow	White or Blue	Black	Green	
Energy Tastes	Bitter	Sweet	Hot & Spicy	Salty	Sour	

Note A: Nerve Tissue, Brain and Spinal Cord are indicated by each of the 5 elements and additionally in the Conception (Ren) and Governing (Du) Vessels. These tissues most closely mimic the direction and flow of energy through meridians, uniting the whole body.

Note B: Blood is also indicated by each of the 5 elements. 'Where Qi Flows, Blood Goes,' is a foundational philosophy of TCM. Looking at the body's Anatomy, nerve fibers run so are they accompanied by blood vessels. This fact underscores the direct relationship between qi and blood.

1: The Pericardium is most closely associated with Dural Tissue. Dural Tissue, like the Pericardial Sac, have similar protective functions providing a fluid-filled enclosure for important organs. Where as Dural Tissue protects the Brain and Spinal Cord, the Pericardium protects the Heart.

2: The Triple Heater is also referred to as the San Jiao and Triple Warmer. With respect to the Triple Heater's function in Traditional Chinese Medicine, it most closely resembles the Hypothalamus and Pituitary Glands of Western Physiology. As such, the Triple Heater has a governing effect upon the endocrine system.

* The Health of the Kidneys are also indicated by the thickness and luster of Head Hair.

** Fascia is the Connective Tissue that envelopes and penetrates each muscle, forming a continuous web commonly referred to as the Myofascial Network. Sinews are Tendons and Ligaments.

Love Pain that became heartache. What happened? My Anatomy started to show the effects of severe and sudden energetic and emotional trauma—head hair falling out (Water Element—fear), paleness (Fire Element—blood vessel damage, Gold Element—no oxygen from shallow breathing), loss of vitality (all elements —fatigue), diagonal cracks in the toenails (Wood and Earth Elements—nail cracks and where they appeared). What was happening to my Physiology? My Physiology had shifted so that my Autonomic Nervous System was in a state of Fight-Or-Flight mode. I didn't know what to do or if anything could be done, but my body had shifted into a protection mode. What was happening to my cellular Biochemistry? I was drained of vitality, literally overnight. It's safe to assume that my cells weren't generating much energy while I was asleep. I was absolutely devastated, and my body showed it.

You see, there are no accidents in the body when you understand what you are looking at. Your body is always providing you with information—even if you don't like what it is saying.

I always wondered what made my toenails crack that night. I didn't know the answer to that question for another six months. I had heard stories of people's hair falling out, but the toenail cracking was weird. Guess what I found out? When I went to school to study *Shiatsu* massage, I learned about meridians. Through the study of meridians—energy fields in the body—I learned that the cracks occurred between two very important points. The Spleen meridian (Earth Element), which is responsible for digesting what goes on in our lives and the Liver meridian (Wood Element), which is connected with frustration. It's no accident that those two toenails cracked. I did not want to swallow or digest what I was told that night. As a result, my body, specifically my Liver (which is one of the body's most emotional organs), felt the enormous burden intensely. It showed up overnight literally through my nails. So that we can go full circle with this, the emotion that surfaced after that was depression.

I was clinically depressed, and also suicidal, for three and a half months. I've had a lot of good times in my life, but those three and a half months were the darkest nights of my soul.

Guess what turned it all around for me? Applying the Cycle of Influencing Energy®.

I began to learn about my body, why my body was doing what it was doing, and how to listen for what it needed. I began to learn how to care for my body. I received Massage Therapy three to four times a week in massage school, which was wonderful. That started to change my anatomical structure. I learned how to breathe and lengthen my body through Yoga, and that healed my physiological functioning. I learned how to eat Organically, and that changed my pH into a much more energy promoting alkaline state. As a result, my body began producing energy again and healing. Believe me, the healing didn't feel good all the time—in fact, sometimes it hurt—but I gave my body what it needed to do what it does best. Together, my body and I healed.

Eventually, my toenails healed, my Heart healed, and my depression went away. I didn't need Paxil, I didn't need Wellbutrin, and I didn't need Prozac. I needed to understand my body. I needed time and support. I needed a healing plan. Fortunately, all of my friends, family, and teachers made all the difference in the world. And during the Healing Process, I developed the Cycle of Influencing Energy® so that I could share something of value so that you can make sense of some of the crazy lessons life presents to you. I hope you will use the information as I have—to create great energy.

The Strength of Natural Medicine

Natural medicine offers a this-makes-sense explanation for why things occur, and a plan for changing them for the better. The beautiful thing about the Cycle of Influencing Energy® is that it provides multiple entry points for you to begin cultivating energy in your body. No matter where you begin, energy will be created throughout each of the five points of the whole system. The greater number of positive lifestyle changes that you make, the more entry points you give yourself as part of the Cycle of Influencing Energy®. Ultimately, these points of entry into healing begin to resonate and develop a wonderful momentum, whereby the energy you're putting into your Healing Process exponentially increases.

As your healing momentum builds, your energy production increases, your emotional state improves, and your body begins to feel undeniably better. As a thought process for healing, the CoIE unifies seemingly divergent philosophies. In conventional medicine a doctor may diagnose you with fatigue or malaise, while a doctor of Traditional Chinese Medicine may diagnose you with Spleen Chi deficiency. The reality for your body is that they're both right. They're both saying the same thing. The CoIE teaches us that the body has many different perspectives with which to assess its health, and that much of the time, different practices of medicine often are saying the same thing in a different way. A Traditional Chinese Medicine doctor may choose to look at your body from a focal point of Energetics, while an allopathic medical doctor may look at your body from a focal point of Anatomy or Physiology. And because they are looking at your body, they can be saying the same thing even if they have different ways of articulating their assessment. But herein lies the strength of Naturopathic Medicine: *Our strength is in our ability to see your body from all of these different points of view simultaneously, and the Cycle of Influencing Energy® is what affords us this wonderful perspective.*

With a functional thought process to work from, you can always continue to add knowledge to it in an organized way. I actually began my professional career as a Mechanical Engineer and later became a Database Developer. So I learned how to organize information. As my passion for natural medicine grew, and as I began to accumulate all this information, I decided that I needed to figure out a way to organize it so that it made sense. And what better way to organize it than from a comprehensive, unified point of view of the body. Naturally, coming from a family of teachers, I had to share this view of healing, how to assess health, and design rock-solid healing plans. So, as fate would have it, I began teaching it to students. Then one night in class it hit me: "Wow, this makes it easy for everybody to understand their own body. Heck, let's use it!" And now I am lucky enough to share this thought process with you.

The strength of natural medicine is that it seldom relies on one therapy to affect a healing response and a healing resolution. Natural medicine at its best utilizes multiple entry points into the Cycle of Influencing Energy® to cultivate the energy necessary to heal. Without energy, the body simply will not heal. Multiple entry points for healing also affords us something else that is essential to the Healing Process—it helps to create the opportunity for participation on your part. To accomplish this, healing plans are designed that utilize the Cycle of Influencing Energy® for assessment and natural therapy selection based on three primary concepts that comprise the **Principle of Advanced Natural Medicine #3**.

FIRST, TREAT THE BODY FROM THE INSIDE OUT.

Expertly address the diet so that food can be medicine, and medicine can be food. There is no greater need for education in our world today than for the education about the human body and how to care for it nutritionally. If you can tell me exactly what Eating Healthy is, then please be my guest. At best, it is a vague concept. At worst, it is misleading marketing propaganda.

SECOND, TREAT THE BODY FROM THE OUTSIDE IN.

With a truly healthy diet, you're putting all these wonderfully nutrient-dense Organic foods, herbs, and supplements into the body. That's a great start. But how about we make that even better? Stimulate the body's innate healing mechanism, the Nervous System. Get touched, get Acupuncture. Receive some natural treatment that stimulates energy flow and the vital forces that course through the body.

THIRD, PARTICIPATE AND MOVE.

Help the first two principles unify in the middle by encouraging participation and movement. The participation may be something as simple as journaling. Or it may involve utilizing the diet as prescribed. There is an undeniable truth in healing naturally—people who move their bodies get better faster. Your body is designed to move—so move it!

Natural Therapy Selection

At our disposal for natural therapy selection are several categories, and this is where my engineering background takes over. The question is, what can we utilize to develop an organized treatment plan so that we can initiate a healing response without creating an overwhelming process? So here, please allow me to share with you my vision for natural therapy organization. I'm sure not every natural therapy available will be listed, but I'm also sure that if one is not listed, you can get an idea about which category it best belongs. There are four categories for natural therapies: Primary Therapies, Complementary Therapies, Fine-Tuning Therapies, and Essential Therapies. Each of these therapeutic categories helps reveal the larger umbrella that is Naturopathic Medicine. When creating a healing plan with multiple points of entry into the Cycle of Influencing Energy®, selecting at least one therapy from each of these four categories typically creates at least four opportunities for cultivation of energy at the Mitochondrial level.

Primary Therapies

A Primary Therapy is one that is most indicated as the lead entry point into the Cycle of Influencing Energy® for energy production. For example, if you twist your ankle, the Primary Therapy isn't clinical nutrition—although that's a good Complementary Therapy. The Primary Therapy is rest. Two weeks later—after the injury has had the time to heal and Scar Tissue has formed—the Primary Therapy becomes Myofascial Massage-Bodywork Therapy, which helps breakdown the Scar Tissue. To initiate any form of therapeutic massage during the inflammatory phase of the Healing Process is to actually get in the way of your body's innate healing capability.

Conversely, let's say you know a friend with a digestive disorder. The Primary Therapy for them isn't Massage-Bodywork Therapy. The Primary Therapy is likely to be clinical nutrition to employ nutrient-dense Organic foods, along with nutrient supplements and botanical medicines, to help heal the root causes of the digestive disorder. Is Massage-Bodywork Therapy an excellent Complementary Therapy? Absolutely—because of its positive effects upon the Autonomic Nervous System. This is a phenomenon I will share with you in detail as we progress. But keep in mind that our pursuit is always the correct natural therapy for the given needs of the body's Healing Process.

In Advanced Natural Medicine, we have at our disposal five basic primary therapies. There is the potential for the addition of more natural therapies in this category, and I hope that the future brings new ones. Still, I am partial to the ones I have selected because of their consistent history of success for my patients and students in practice. Primary Therapies include:

1. **ORGANIC CLINICAL NUTRITION**—Eat your way to health. Let food be your medicine, and your medicine be your food. These are great ideas that have a ton of wisdom within them. And what better way to turn food into medicine than with pure, clean foods that support your body and the environment? If we embellish this concept to learn exactly which foods support your Immune System and that should become staples of your diet, then we're really playing with some power. Organic Clinical Nutrition includes lifestyle, diet, supplementation, and botanical medicines, or herbs.

2. **DETOXIFICATION—TWENTY-EIGHT-DAY CELLULAR CLEANSING®**—A clean body performs better than a body saddled with environmental pollution, infections, and dietary

excesses. Strategies for detoxification are among the strongest known preventative medicines.

3. **MASSAGE-BODYWORK—RELEASE POINT THERAPY®**—Welcome to the healing power of therapeutic touch. Skilled hands can do as much for your body as any scalpel or surgery. All therapeutic touch accomplishes at least one positive goal—the activation of the Parasympathetic Rest and Digest division of your body's Autonomic Nervous System. In other words, therapeutic touch helps you digest your food and sleep better, leading to a much more effective Immune System.

4. **IV NUTRIENTS AND CHELATION THERAPY**—Sometimes the body's digestion is too depleted. Sometimes the body is in immediate need of nutrients. And sometimes the body is in need of detoxifying heavy metals accumulated in the deeper tissues. In these situations, IV administration of pH-balanced nutrients and/or chelating agents can completely reverse a disease process.

5. **YOGA**—People who move their bodies regularly while sweating heal faster. After a decade of working with Yoga communities, I can come to no other conclusions about this amazing healing modality. Of course, Yoga is so much more than the awkward body positions and funny-sounding breathing that marketing often reduces it to. Yoga does something better than any other movement-based exercise modality—it creates space as it creates strength. Space, movement, energy. And a strong body ultimately becomes a strong mind.

Quick Note: Why Twenty-Eight Days?

The natural healer's job is to create a positive shift in the health of the patient as quickly as possible. By utilizing the five primary therapies in the correct situations, a positive shift can be achieved within the Cycle of Influencing Energy® quickly. Remember that for whatever reason, your body is designed to heal in twenty-eight-day cycles. The Naturopathic Physician's job is to decide which therapies are going to give that patient the greatest positive shift within the first twenty-eight days of treatment. Experience teaches that a patient who feels a positive shift in his or her health within twenty-eight days is likely to stay on course with the full treatment plan, and as a result, see the Healing Process through to the healing resolution.

If I can't help a patient feel a positive shift within twenty-eight days, I know that there is a strong likelihood that the patient will lose faith in me, and perhaps in natural medicine altogether. I just can't sleep well at night with that, so I typically push the envelope in the first month to ensure that we have done everything possible within the patient's abilities and what they are able to afford. But it all starts with listening to best determine the obstacles to cure and from there, selecting the Primary Therapy. When this is done well, natural medicine is incredibly successful and wonderful to be a part of.

Complementary Therapies

Complementary Therapies are those that are going to best support the Primary Therapy and create more entry points into the Cycle of Influencing Energy® for healing. They are going to complement the primary therapy to help create the desired healing outcome without becoming overwhelming. A Complementary Therapy can be any of the following:

1. **ANY PRIMARY THERAPY, FINE-TUNING THERAPY, OR ESSENTIAL THERAPY**

2. **SAUNA THERAPY**—Used for thousands of years to assist in the detoxification of the whole body through the body's largest organ—the Skin. Sweating is a gentle medicinal way of lowering the loads of environmental pollutants, as was rediscovered for our brave firefighters following September 11, 2001. Saunas also have proven to

be effective in reversing Congestive Heart Failure. Of all the types of Sauna Therapy, Infrared Saunas are the most recommended for their ability to also kill infections in the soft tissues.

3. **HYDROTHERAPY**—Also known as Water Cure Hydrotherapy originally was utilized to create temperature differences in the body to better activate the Immune System, and to stimulate blood flow in affected areas of injured tissue. When you think of Hydrotherapy, think of alternating heat and cold treatments.

4. **PRANAYAMA, TAI CHI, AND QI GONG BREATHING PRACTICES**—The art of breathing at its finest. Breathing practices afford the practitioner the opportunity to saturate the body with alkalizing and energy supporting oxygen. That these practices promote a mastery over emotions and the physical body is simply an amazing bonus.

5. **ORGANIC JUICE FASTING**—The art of fasting without fasting. Organic Juice Fasting, in spite of its name, is technically not fasting due to the availability of carbohydrates that support energy production. Nevertheless, Organic Juice Fasting is a way to deliver a medicinal amount of nutrients to your cells almost as quickly as a Nutrient IV.

6. **MASSAGE THERAPY**—So what's the difference between Massage Therapy and Massage-Bodywork Therapy? The skill set of the practitioner. Licensed Massage Practitioners undoubtedly display a higher skill set, knowledge base, and touch sensitivity than entry-level Massage Therapists. That said, nothing beats a good massage after a tough day. All healing touch is good touch. My personal favorites includes *Shiatsu*, Reflexology, *Lomi Lomi*, Thai Massage, and *Watsu* to name just a few.

7. **SPINAL MOBILIZATION**—Spinal Mobilization is an excellent Complementary Therapy for restoring the space necessary for optimal postural alignment and assisting nerve conduction throughout the spinal cord and entire body. Spinal Mobilization includes the use of inversion tables.

8. **AUTHENTIC EXERCISE REGIMENS LIKE P90X®, PILATES, MARTIAL ARTS, AND DANCE**—Muscle confusion is a term that was coined by P90X® creator Tony Horton. The idea of mixing up exercise regimens so that you continually challenge your body with each routine is a phenomenal experience. That it is done with such encouragement as is often found with Pilates teachers is the energetic bonus. What I've often found interesting in my work is that martial artists and dancers have the tendency to move the most energy throughout their bodies. This is a phenomenon I have only been able to attribute to the repetition of specific motions that are coordinated with breath. The practice of Martial Arts, Dance, and Yoga create more space in the body for energy flow, while using breath that is coordinated with movement to accelerate energy throughout the body's natural energy channels.

9. **SINUS IRRIGATION**—Cleaning out the nose is essential for optimal breathing, and thus, optimal energy production. This is a great treatment from the inside out.

10. **CLAY PACKS, HERBAL WRAPS, AND MINERAL BATHS**—Sometimes it's just nice to have that spa-pampered feeling. From a medicinal standpoint, spa days help care for the largest organ of the body—the Skin.

11. **MINDFULNESS PRACTICES AND JOURNALING**—You are where your thoughts are—this is one of the basic tenets of a mindfulness practice, which helps you focus on the present moment. Journaling is a reflective practice that helps you sort through thoughts that can take you away from the present moment, and lock you into the destructive habits of your past.

Fine-Tuning Therapies

Fine-Tuning Therapies—like the name implies—are a category of natural therapies designed to tune the body similar to how a musical instrument is tuned. So let's embellish upon this analogy. If we look at the body as a musical instrument, say a guitar, then certainly it will play better after it is tuned. However, let's imagine that the body of the guitar is warped, damaged, and twisted. Imagine that the neck of the guitar is broken. No matter how hard you try to tune the strings of the damaged guitar, the instrument will never achieve its true beautiful sound. Such is the similarity with the human body and the use of Fine-Tuning Therapies. *Fine-Tuning Therapies are most effective after some level of health and energy production have been restored within the body.* Fine-Tuning Therapies are going to be most effective once the guitar body has regained its ideal physical structure—in other words, once the Anatomy has achieved its ideal alignment. With energy present, Fine-Tuning Therapies can help overcome healing plateaus. Fine-Tuning Therapies can help take the Healing Process to the next level. Fine-Tuning Therapies include:

1. **HOMEOPATHY**—Created by Dr. Samuel Hahnemann during the late 1700s. Homeopathic remedies are able to take the energy signature of a substance theoretically based on fixed hydrogen-bonding structures to create changes in cellular DNA responses to the remedy. Homeopathy is the art of curing, based on resemblances or similarities. The principle is that every disease is curable by medicines that are diluted in concentrations near or below Avogadro's Number. Avogadro's Number is the limit of dilutions at which no active ingredients currently exist from the original solution. Therefore, solutions that have been diluted beyond 6.0221415×10^{23} exceed Avogadro's Number. While there are a substantial number of medical skeptics that dispute the 'science' of this natural therapy, there are also approximately 430 million people worldwide who subscribe to it. I suppose it's possible to fool 430 million people throughout the world... In a healthy person, the level of concentration should produce symptoms similar to those that characterize the specific disease.

2. **ACUPUNCTURE**—First recorded as a therapeutic modality more than thirty-five hundred years ago during the Shang Dynasty. Acupuncture stimulates energy pathways throughout the body that originates from the body's individual organs as a way of homeostatic balance. Acupuncture acts to improve energy production and the health of the organs.

3. **CLINICAL WATER FASTING**—Both a physical and spiritual practice designed to give the majority of your body's organs time off to rid themselves of accumulated toxins and excess. In doing so, the physical body becomes a conduit for a spiritual experience.

4. **MEDITATION**—Mindfulness amplified for the ultimate peace of mind. What's always interesting is that many people attempt Meditation with a damaged or ailing body. A person has to prepare for Meditation through proper care of the body if they want to realize its benefits and sustain the practice.

5. **NATIVE AMERICAN SWEAT LODGES**—Is there a difference between Sauna Therapy and Native American Sweat Lodges? Absolutely. Like any Fine-Tuning Therapy, Native American Sweat have the ability to reach the spiritual body.

6. **CRANIOSACRAL THERAPY**—Developed by Dr. John Upledger as a way to access the Parasympathetic Rest and Digest division of the Autonomic Nervous System without force. It is a beautiful therapy that is often categorized as massage, but in truth, it is so much more.

7. **PRAYER**—Hopefully, this needs no explanation.

Essential Therapies

Essential Therapies are the most affordable, cost-effective natural therapies, and yet, they are the most easily overlooked and dismissed. Let's see—Essential Therapies are free, easy, and they make a huge difference during the Healing Process. Yep—all good reasons to dismiss their effectiveness. Essential Therapies include the following:

1. **POSITIVE INTERNAL DIALOGUE**—Positive Internal Dialogue is the way that you speak to yourself. Are you encouraging and supportive? Or are you harsh and judgmental? Essential Therapies are founded on three beliefs that I want to share with you. First, it is essential to encourage everyone, including—and especially—yourself. It is essential to be encouraging at all times because we hear discouraging words too frequently throughout our typical every day. Second, it is essential to be disciplined so that you can develop consistency for optimal results. And third, it is essential to believe that you can *and will* heal. People who believe they will heal tend to heal fantastically well. This is the ultimate foundation for all Essential Therapies—Positive Internal Dialogue based on self-encouragement, discipline, and belief.

2. **SLEEP**—Sleep is essential because it is during rest that your Immune System is most active. If you are intent on healing, understand that your body requires a minimum of seven to eight hours of uninterrupted sleep. The scientific explanation, which will be discussed in greater detail later, involves cellular replication and cellular detoxification. I can already hear some of you saying: "I have so much work to do, kids, and so many responsibilities. How am I supposed to get seven to eight hours of sleep?"

   Your body needs sleep. If you can't get continuous sleep, then there are other options that can help you. One option is to take beauty naps during the day. Naps work for children, the senior population, those in Latin American countries, and they also can work for you. Another option is one of my favorites. At least one day each week, let yourself wake up when your body is ready to wake up. No alarms. No schedules. Just you waking when your body says it's ready to go. If that turns out to be ten hours or more, so be it.

3. **SUNLIGHT**—Sunlight provides energy and strengthens your vital force. Sunlight also is essential for helping your body manufacture Vitamin D, which we have learned has an important role to play in your Immune System's health. Vitamin D is essential—along with Vitamin K, Calcium, and Magnesium—for building optimal bone density. Did you know that sunlight also helps regulate reproductive hormones—especially in the female body—and that it builds healthy levels of mood-stabilizing neurotransmitters like Serotonin?

   Depending on your Skin color and eye color, you will need approximately forty percent of your Skin exposed to sunlight—or to full-spectrum lightbulbs in your office or home—for your body to manufacture Vitamin D. Naturally, if you

Safe Sunlight	Skin Type	Skin Tone and Eye Color	Tanning Behavior
10 minutes	1	Fair Skin—Blue, Green, Hazel Eyes	Always Burns
20 minutes	2	Light Skin—Blue, Green, Hazel Eyes	Often Burns
30 minutes	3	Light Skin—Hazel, Brown Eyes	Usually Tans
40 minutes	4	Olive Skin—Hazel, Brown Eyes	Often Tans
50 minutes	5	Caramel Skin—Brown, Dark Brown Eyes	Always Tans
60 minutes	6	Black Skin—Dark Brown Eyes	N/A

are using environmentally friendly sunscreen or exposing less of your Skin to the sunlight, then you will need more time in the sun for your body to manufacture Vitamin D. (See Safe Sunlight Chart on previous page.)

4. **CLEAN WATER**—Your body is two-thirds to three-quarters water, depending on your health and age. So making sure that you're taking in enough clean water is essential to the Healing Process. Without getting too deep into a twenty-first century problem, understand that Tap Water—even with a Reverse Osmosis (RO) System—will not get the job done for your body. Tap Water often contains the following obstacles that can stand in the way of healing: Lead, Aluminum, Sodium Fluoride, Bacteria and Viruses, Chlorine, Chloroform, Methyl-t-butyl ether (MTBE)-Rocket Fuel, Pesticides, Treated and Filtered Wastewater, Antibiotics, Antidepressants, Blood Pressure Medications, and more. Now the problem with this is that each of these factors contributes to fatigue, diminished cellular performance, and stunted cellular growth.

   Safe Bottled Water, as determined by the National Resources Defense Council, makes the most sense for consumption. Your body is made up of a large percentage of water, so make it clean water. At the time of this writing, the following companies tested safe for their water's purity: Ice Age®, Hawaiian Springs®, FIJI®, Naya®, Crystal Geyser®, Arrowhead®, DASANI®, Aquafina®, Evian®, San Pellegrino®, and smartwater®.

5. **CLEAN AIR**—Depending on where you live, clean air is either easy or difficult to obtain. If you live in a major metropolitan area that is located in a valley, clean air may be difficult to come by. What you can control regardless of where you live, however, is your home. Clean air in the home does very well, with attention to a few details: 1) Make sure your home is filled with plants that purify the air. These include cactuses, devil's ivy, and dark green leaf foliages. 2) If you have a central heating and air conditioning unit, make sure that you use a Minimum Efficiency Reporting Value (MERV) eight or higher-rated air filter. 3) Make sure your air filters are replaced at least four to six times per year. 4) Open your windows whenever possible. 5) Keep in mind that flooring can make all the difference. Use of hardwood, tile, or stained concrete—*particularly in the bedroom*—can reduce allergen accumulation by more than 90 percent when compared to carpeting. If you value healthy air, remove carpeting from your home.

6. **LAUGHTER**—This may be one of my most favorite prescriptions to write. It is definitely in the same category as taking a well-deserved vacation from negativity and complaining. Laughter is medicine for the psyche, as well as the Autonomic Nervous System. Laughter promotes healthy expression that help alleviate accumulated stress on the nerves. If you take life too seriously, you'll probably miss a good laugh.

7. **CONSISTENT PRACTICE OF YOUR BELIEF SYSTEM**—I teach a very special set of humanitarian principles that have been handed down for literally five thousand years. What I love about these principles is that you can often find them embedded within most existing belief systems. They are not religious, but they do work in accord with all religions of the world. They apply to all genders, socioeconomic conditions, and ages. I stated earlier that Positive Internal Dialogue is an Essential Therapy founded upon self-encouragement, discipline, and belief. It is essential to remind yourself of what you believe every day, *before* you leave the security of your home and family and venture out into this breakneck-paced world we have created. Knowing who you are and exactly what you are about makes decision-making remarkably easy, regardless of the situation. When in doubt, you can safely call on your beliefs to guide you with refreshing, absolute certainty. This act will consistently help you cultivate energy. I don't know about you, but that makes me feel all warm and fuzzy inside.

Regardless of the beliefs that you hold dear to your heart as definitions for right and wrong, the only way to practice them consistently is with courage and daily repetition. Without courage and daily repetition there can be no consistency, and your decision-making and the results that follow will take you on a roller coaster ride. Courage and daily practice give you the skills to get off the roller coaster at your leisure, helping to empower you. That's right—you don't have to live at the mercy of your own life.

If you are ready to end the negative cycles of influencing energy that life may be presenting to you, then I offer these principles for your consideration: *No harm, truth, no stealing, continence (positive thoughts, words, deeds), compassion, forgiveness, endurance, humility, cleanliness, and moderate healthy diet.* There are ten additional humanitarian principles that work to strengthen the first ten. This second group includes: *Austerity (strict discipline), appreciation, modesty, charity, sacrifice, discernment (knowing right from wrong for you), repetition of healthy habits, celebration of your Higher Power, listening to your heart (gut instinct), and trusting and believing in the perfection of life.*

Cycle of Influencing Energy®—Final Thoughts

When we draw natural therapies from each of the four categories—Primary Therapies, Complementary Therapies, Fine-Tuning Therapies, and Essential Therapies—to design a treatment plan, each provides multiple, synergistic entry points into the Cycle of Influencing Energy® to create energy and a positive shift in health. A treatment plan that is designed using these principles creates the most ideal situation for you and others you work with to experience a restoration of health.

Example: Craving Flavor: **Salty**

Energetic Stimulated: Fire Earth Metal **Water** Wood

Attempted Energy-Cultivating Response: **Trust, Belief, Faithfulness**

1. Craving Flavor: ____________________

Energetic Stimulated: Fire Earth Metal Water Wood

Attempted Energy-Cultivating Response: ____________________

2. Craving Flavor: ____________________

Energetic Stimulated: Fire Earth Metal Water Wood

Attempted Energy-Cultivating Response: ____________________

3. Craving Flavor: ____________________

Energetic Stimulated: Fire Earth Metal Water Wood

Attempted Energy-Cultivating Response: ____________________

4. Craving Flavor: ____________________

Energetic Stimulated: Fire Earth Metal Water Wood

Attempted Energy-Cultivating Response: ____________________

Listening To Your Amazing Body

Believe it or not, your body will tell you what it needs—often through cravings for certain foods or flavors. Understand that when your body craves a particular flavor, it is attempting to stimulate the Energetic that the flavor corresponds with. For example, craving something sweet is an attempt to stimulate the Earth Energetic, and along with it, Energy-Cultivating Responses for rational decision-making and a calm, clear mind.

For at least one day, write down every flavor craving that you have. Then use the Five-Element Energetics Chart (See **Figure 2.2**) to learn which Energetic your body is attempting to stimulate, and which Energy-Cultivating Response it is working to utilize.

What You Can Do To Cultivate Energy Today

If you find that you are craving certain flavors—like sweet—then it is best to choose one that does not take you from a deficient to excess state. The tendency to overindulge often happens when we crave something sweet, but seek highly refined sugar that is in sodas, candies, and energy drinks.

RESOLUTION #2

Choose a new sweet. When you find yourself craving something sweet, select an Organic healthy sweet like a fruit or a vegetable to stimulate your Earth Energy. After a week or two of choosing natural sweets, you'll find that your taste buds will adjust, and that you will discover new flavors in these Organic foods that will help to stabilize your emotional states throughout the day.

Design a sample healing plan for yourself. Select one natural therapeutic from each category. For example, select one Primary Therapy, two Complementary Therapies, one Fine-Tuning Therapy, and one Essential Therapy from the lists of organized natural therapies in this chapter.

RESOLUTION #3

For two weeks, put your healing plan into action by utilizing your Primary Therapy and Essential Therapy every day, and by utilizing both your Complementary Therapy and Fine-Tuning Therapy at least twice during the fourteen-day trial. Take pictures of your entire body and your face before the trial, and at the end of the trial.

HEALING JOURNAL RECORDING

Using your Healing Journal, record your moods, thoughts, and positive experiences with the new healthy sweet you have selected. Also record the design of your healing plan, why you chose those therapies, and your moods, thoughts, and positive experiences during the fourteen-day trial.

Additional Ideas for Making Positive Changes

What can you do today to cultivate energy in your life? I would say the best recommendation that I can give you is to complete this book and the activities within it. I have purposely loaded this book with useful information so that you can use it as a reference guide for years to come. So don't feel like you have to remember everything, as that's not the point. Take what you need from this information, and apply it to your life.

Make as many changes as your enthusiasm will allow without feeling overwhelmed. Also keep in mind that one positive change at a time will still be realized throughout your whole body, so there is not necessarily a rush to try it all at once.

If you're dealing with a serious or moderately serious health issue, and you're looking for help, I would invite you to give Naturopathic Medicine and her wonderful licensed physicians a try. We are ready to listen to you, and to take interest in your story. We are ready to help you feel important in the way that you deserve to feel important. To find a solid Naturopathic Physician, go to www.naturopathic.org and find a qualified and eager-to-help ND.

Good Luck!

CHAPTER 3: THE 4 CONSIDERATIONS FOR HEALING

How Your Body Perceives Stress

Interesting Insights to look for in this chapter:

- What being ticklish reveals about stress from Emotional Charge.
- Every dollar spent on Organic foods is a vote cast for your future.
- How activating your feet can make your back feel better.
- What a beaver's dam has to do with energy flow.

Principle of Advanced Natural Medicine #4:

Your body does not differentiate between various types of stress. Stress from internalized emotion causes just as much cellular damage as stress from acidic diets. The body responds to all stresses in similar fashion, by garnering its Energetic resources to initiate a proactive healing response involving the Immune System.

Stress Is Much More Than An Unpaid Bill

Under any stress, your body becomes more susceptible to infection. From your body's perspective stress, is anything that results in cellular damage. Can emotional reactions be stressful? Of course they can. But what about a can of soda, or the chemicals in our food supply? What about a slumping body posture or previous injuries from which we still feel the effects? These are a few of the many of ways that your body perceives stress. Understand that your body has little concern for what is causing the stressful damage, but a tremendous concern for how to heal once the damage is done. When the amount of stress held in the body exceeds the body's ability to produce energy, disease can be the only outcome.

Your body's number one job is to promote the continuance of life. Thus, the Nervous System has been pre-wired to launch a Healing Process, regardless of the cause of damage. Your body's job is to heal. So let's explore the basics of this process at the cellular level.

If even one of your cells experiences a stressful situation and becomes damaged, what is the first thing that occurs? The perception of the damage. Without the perception of damage—often felt as a pain signal—your body cannot know that a cell is injured and in need of attention. So pain serves a very useful purpose because it initiates the healing response. What happens next? After a pain signal is sent and received, your body launches into action and coordinates the Nervous System, Cardiovascular System, and especially your Immune System.

In classical texts, wound healing often is modeled in such a way that there are only four stages of healing—Inflammation, Migration, Proliferation, and Maturation. So I ask you: What initiated the whole process? Damage and the perception of damage. Before inflammation can serve its essential purpose—which is to drive blood, oxygen, and nutrients into the affected area—the body must first know where to target healing response. With pain helping to identify the exact location of the damage, immune cells can migrate to the area and multiply—a process also known as proliferation. Yes, that's correct. *All healing—whether it be from an infection, the detoxification of environmental pollution, or even a routine injury—requires a healthy and efficient Immune System.* This is a major aspect of the Sophisticated Simplicity we have been talking about. Once the area has been cleared and cleaned by the immune cells, Scar Tissue is formed to help reinforce the area. Because Scar Tissue also limits range of motion, it can be a major reason why rehabilitation can be so difficult following surgery or an injury.

Most bodies are stressed out, and therefore, acidic. Due to this fact, most Healing Processes end with a significant amount of Scar Tissue still present within the soft tissues. Thankfully, it doesn't have to be this way. With the help of an alkaline environment for optimal energy production, your body can produce enough enzymes to help breakdown excess Scar Tissue. Enzymes allow your body to effectively remodel the previously injured area in order to maximize space, movement, and tensile strength. The goal of the body's Healing Process is to return the damaged area to as close to 100 percent of the pre-injured state as possible.

So, what we are proposing here is that there are several additional steps to the Sophisticated Simplicity of a proactive healing response (**Additional steps in bold**):

1. **Pain response resulting from cellular damage.**
2. Inflammation leading to the activation of the Immune System.
3. Migration of immune cells into the affected area.
4. Proliferation of immune cells within the affected area to accelerate healing.
5. Maturation of Scar Tissue (myofascial adhesions) to reinforce the affected area.
6. **Breakdown of excess Scar Tissue to optimize space, movement, and energy production.**
7. **Final remodeling of the affected area.**

Most classical texts ignore the pain response as a necessary part of the Healing Process, and exclude altogether the final breakdown of the Scar Tissue as an essential and final stage of wound healing. Yet the take home message remains the same. Stress leads to cellular damage, and once the damage has been perceived, your body employs the same step-by-step process of Sophisticated Simplicity each and every time. It is this seven-step process that allows your body to ignore the cause of the damage, and instead, focus on the task of healing.

So then the real question becomes: Is pain a bad thing? No—it is an essential thing. And is inflammation a bad thing? No—it is essential for the Immune System to do its job effectively. *Take away pain, and take away inflammation, and what you are left with is a very ineffective healing response that leaves the affected tissue ripe for infection, pollution deposition, and re-injury.* But isn't that what we are doing far too frequently with the advent of pain medications and anti-inflammatory pills? I have some good information for you about the effects of medications when we get to the chapter on the Immune System. You are going to love that chapter!

So when damage doesn't heal, what are the usual causes? Look no further than deficiencies in energy, deficiencies in nutrient resources, and an excess of substances blocking the aforementioned seven-step process.

What is the purpose of pain? What is your body saying with the help of pain? Your body is saying that damage is occurring at the cellular level. The more intense the pain, the greater the damage—and often, to more immediately critical functions. That's what we know about pain.

So what is your body saying with inflammation? Inflammation is your body's attempt to inform you that it is healing the damaged cells, creating space for energy to flow again. And if the pain and inflammation are chronic, what do we know then? When pain and inflammation are chronic, the inescapable truth is that damage is reoccurring. The pursuit for the healer's inquiring mind is why—what is causing the damage? For an answer to this last question, I present the 4 Considerations for Healing.

The 4 Considerations for Healing

Sodas and previous injuries are seldom answers I hear in response to the question, what stresses you out? I seldom hear things like lack of sleep or forgetting to breathe from the diaphragm. Do you know why? Because we haven't been taught what the body perceives as stressful. In fact, what your body experiences as stress is much more diverse than emotion. That said, never underestimate the power or potency of emotion as a stressor or healer. What your body views as stressful becomes what we term in Naturopathic Medicine as obstacles to cure. Obstacles to cure can be organized into the following 4 Considerations for Healing (See **Figure 3.1**) as follows:

1. Emotional Charge
2. Acidic Cellular Environments
3. Biomechanical Misalignments
4. Scar Tissue (Myofascial Adhesions)

The 4 Considerations for Healing is a way to categorize any stress your body may experience. As obstacles to cure, if we understand stress correctly, and if we use the Cycle of Influencing Energy® to create entry points for Mitochondria to produce energy, then we can effectively turn a chronic degenerative process into a positive Healing Process.

The 4 Considerations for Healing

Sources of Stress that Create Obstacles to Cure

1 Emotional Charge

~ Create Energy Draining Holes in the Auric Fields & Disruptions of Meridian Flow

~ With Meridian Flow Disrupted Nerve, Immune, Endocrine, Heart, and Digestive Function Suffer

2 Acidic Cellular Environments

~ Blood - Acidic Substances that have accumulated in the body over recent months, are being circulated, and hopefully eliminated

~ Tissue - Acidic Substances that have accumulated since conception and may be bound within the deeper tissues

~ Consider Nutrient Deficiencies, Industrialized Fast Foods, Environmental Pollutions & Energy Draining Reactions leading to Suppressed Immunity and subsequent Chronic Infections (Bacterial, Yeast, Viral, Parasitic)

3 Biomechanical Misalignments

~ Sub-Optimal Postures that impede diaphragmatic breathing and unnecessarily consume energy, by forcing muscles to overwork thus placing a great physical burden upon joints, ligaments, and tendons leaving them susceptible to injury

4 Scar Tissue

~ Physical Injuries from Accidents (Automobile, Sports-Related, Surgeries, Repetitive Use like Carpal Tunnel, Etc.)

~ Internal Injury from Acidic Cellular Environments (Please see Item 2)

~ Reoccurring Injury from Sub-Optimal Biomechanical Alignment (Please See Item 3)

~ Internalized Unexpressed Emotions, Often Self-Inflicted Injury to the Spirit (Please See Item 1)

Genesis Health Systems

Figure 3.1

Emotional Charge— Are You Ticklish?

WHAT IS IT? Emotional Charge is literally bioelectric charging of the Nervous System. Your Nervous System is truly amazing—it is responsible for perceiving, processing, and responding to any and all stimuli. The average adult Nervous System is comprised of approximately one thousand billion individual neurons, and each neuron is comprised of three parts—an axon, a cell body, and multiple dendrites (See **Figure 3.2**). The axon sends a bioelectric signal from the cell body, launching all movement. The cell body processes the summary of signals coming from the dendrites, which is an amazing testament to the typical cell body, which can receive between one thousand and ten thousand signals simultaneously. The dendrites receive all the signals from either stimulus or preceding axons. The dendrites play an instrumental role in the neuron's ability to reach the bioelectric potential necessary to send the signal through the axon. The process of surpassing the bioelectric potential necessary to send a signal along the axon is known as threshold.

Let's consider a simple example to illustrate this concept. It takes 99 millivolts for a neuron to reach threshold, and to have enough charge to launch energy through its axon. So let's say that we have one dendrite that accumulates a charge of 100 millivolts. This stimulus reaches threshold and will launch energy through the axon. Let's also say for comparison that we have four dendrites that each are accumulating 25 millivolts of charge. This is enough combined stimulus to reach threshold, and enough to launch energy through the axon. Let's finally say that we have 100 dendrites that each are accumulating 1 millivolt of charge. Again, this is enough combined stimulus to reach threshold, and to therefore launch energy through the axon. The last fact to take away from the discussion of this process is that dendrites have the ability to accumulate and remember previous stimulus. The application of this information is that a dendrite can retain memory of previous events and *pre-charge* itself in anticipation of a reaction or response to a perceived stimulus. This is the exact premise upon which all learned behaviors are established, and it provides us with a rational explanation for the phenomenon of being ticklish.

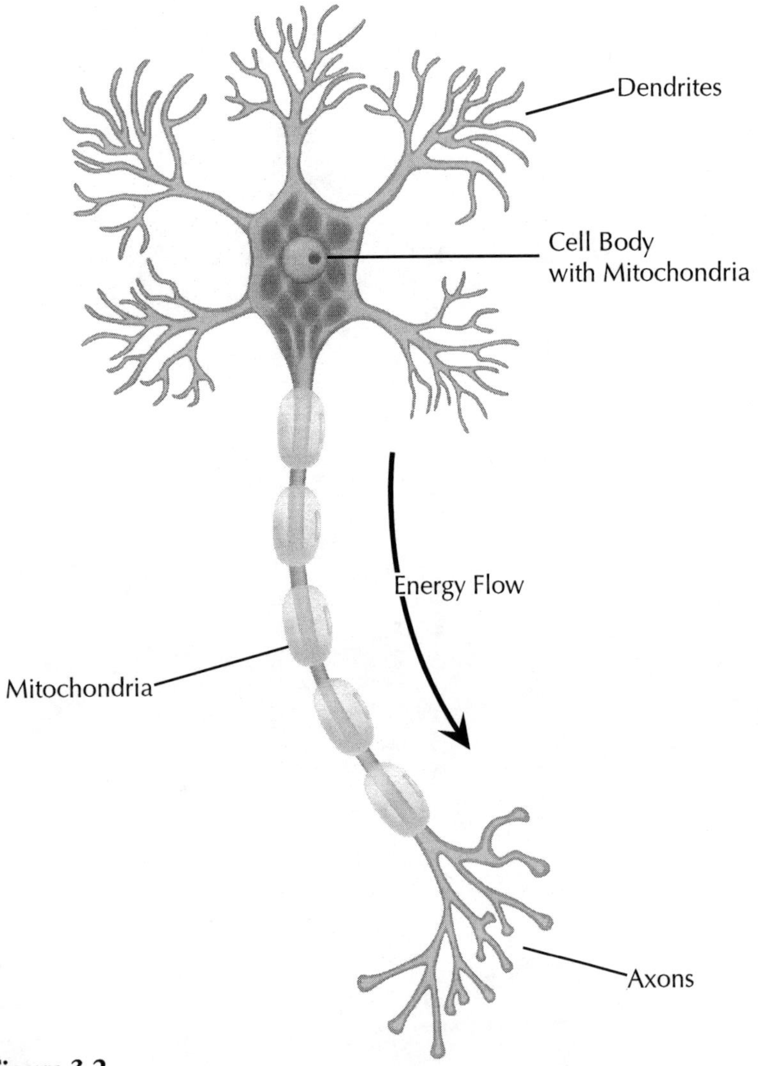

Figure 3.2
Emotional Charge builds upon the dendrites. The more Emotional Charge the more easily threshold is crossed and a signal sent through the axon. This is ticklishness in adults.

A single neuron can have between one thousand and ten thousand dendrites but requires only 70 millivolts to reach threshold. Remember that each of these dendrites has memory, and that their accumulation of bioelectric charge has the ability to surpass the 70 millivolts necessary to exceed threshold. If we say that the threshold in a calm body is 70 millivolts, and that the stress of Emotional Charge lowers the bioelectric energy necessary to attain threshold, then we are saying that stress pre-charges the Nervous System in a way that makes it easier for a signal to reach threshold. This gives a whole new meaning to the phrase getting on your nerves, and perhaps explains why one might overreact. For example, a person with a moderate to high content of Emotional Charge on their dendrites can take their optimal threshold of 70 millivolts down to 40 millivolts. Because the new threshold is much lower than the optimal threshold, this person will have less room for error because it takes less stimulus to produce an energy surge through the axon. So what does this have to do with being ticklish?

Your body is a wonderful example of design and efficiency. How might an adult know that they are carrying too much Emotional Charge on their Nervous System? The answer is being ticklish at specify energy points on the front and back of their body (See **Figure 3.3**). Think about being ticklish. Typically it's a very light and/or quick touch to specific areas of the body that creates a pull-away retraction, a knocking away of the offending hand, and perhaps a little laughter. How could such a light stimulus create such a dramatic effect? Threshold has been lowered, and as a result, less stimulus is needed to create a reaction. *The more ticklish a person is, the lower their threshold, and the more pre-charged their Nervous System.*

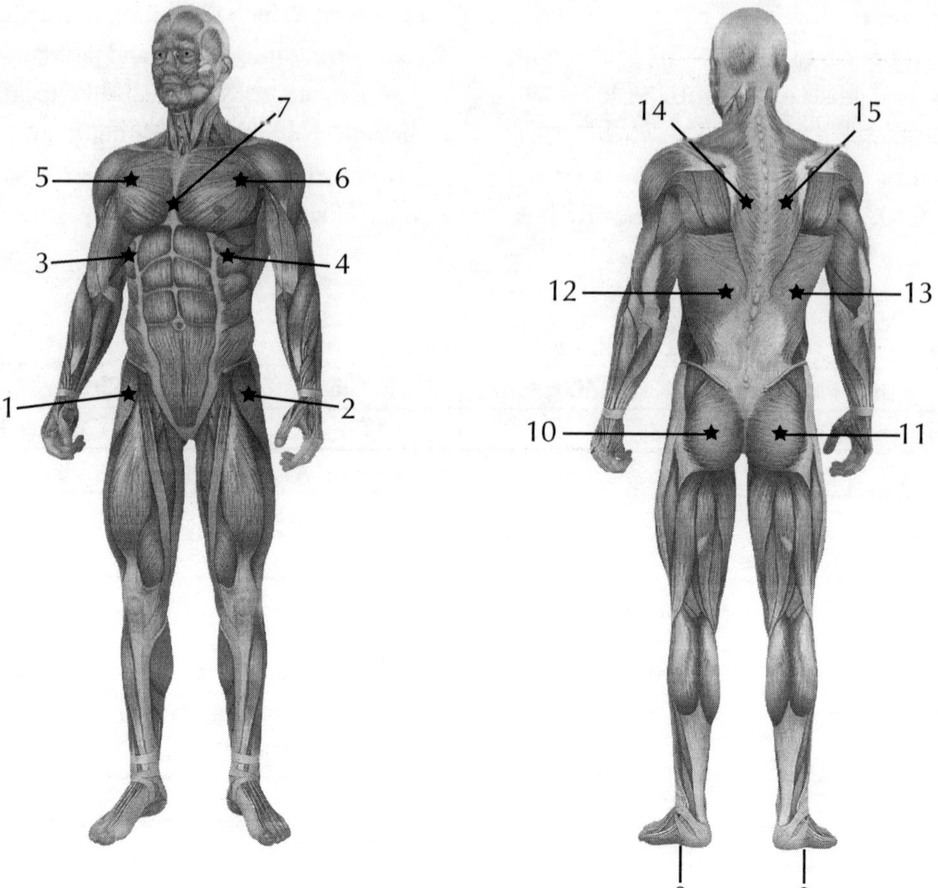

Figure 3.3
Remember that the front of the body reveals what's going on between the person and their world, while the back of the body reveals what's going on between the person and themselves.

Now believe it or not, where a person is ticklish can tell us a great deal about what is creating the Emotional Charge, and as a result, how to lower their threshold. On the front of the body, there are seven high charge points, while on the back of the body there are eight high charge points, including the feet. In an effort to simplify this information, consult the table below with this knowledge. High charge points correspond with specific meridian points of Traditional Chinese Medicine. High charge points on the front of the body reveal what's going on between you and your world. High charge points on the back of the body reveal what's going on internally between you and yourself.

Can you check these high charge points on your own? No—the most accurate reading will come from a practitioner checking them for you and monitoring your reaction on a scale of 0 to 10. A reaction that is reported as ticklish or painful, but in which there is no retraction of the body or change in facial expression, would be a 1 to 3 out of 10. A reaction that is reported as ticklish or painful and in which there is mild retraction of the body, twitching, or change in facial expression, would be given a rating of 4 to 6 out of 10. A reaction that is reported as ticklish or painful, and in which there is moderate to severe retraction of the body, twitching, and change in facial expression, would be rated between 7 and 10 out of 10. At which high charge point this activation occurs reveals what is *potentially* the underlying cause of the Emotional Charge. The higher the charge, the more likely that Emotional Charge is a significant obstacle to cure.

HOW IS IT CREATED?

Emotional Charge is the result of unexpressed emotion or emotion that has not been resolved through satisfying outcome. Laugh out loud and the whole world laughs with you, but when you cry, you cry alone. When emotion is internalized, it's damaging and painful. It is so important to say what you want to say, when you want to say it, AND in a way that it can be received. This is the great skill in all communication, and it can require a tremendous amount of creativity, timing, attention, and redirection of energy. Why be consumed by anger when you can transform it into humor and get the desired outcome? Just a thought. Would you like to know if you have developed a habit of holding your tongue but don't have anyone to tickle you? Yes? Great—let's look to your body for the answer.

Front of the Body—Between You and Your World

High Charge Points	Corresponding Meridian Point	Likely Cause of Emotional Charge
1 and 2	Stomach 31	Sexual Frustration or Trauma, Creative Block
3 and 4	Liver 14	Frustration, Anger, Lack of Confidence
5 and 6	Lung 1	Prolonged Sadness
7	Conception 17	Deep Love Pain, Heartache

Back of the Body—Between You and Yourself

High Charge Points	Corresponding Meridian Point	Likely Cause of Emotional Charge
8 and 9	Kidney 1	Apprehension Moving Forward in Life, Doubt, Fear
10 and 11	Gall Bladder 30	Not Flexible Enough In Opinions, Sexually Repressed
12 and 13	Urinary Bladder 47	Frustrated, Impatient, Angry with Self
14 and 15	Urinary Bladder 45	Overly Protective, Abused, Closed Heart

If you feel underneath your jawbone and in front of your throat, you'll feel through the Skin where your tongue originates. Press into and gently squeeze this region (See **Figure 3.4**). If this area feels hard or tense, your body is telling you that you are holding your tongue tightly, and that you are withholding your true thoughts and expressions. You are withholding speaking your mind and speaking your truth. You can easily establish a point of reference to determine whether your tongue is tight or not. Find someone who's outspoken (and a non-smoker), and feel underneath their jawbone. Feel a difference? Or find a dog or cat and feel under their jawbone—feel how loose and fluid the muscles are underneath?

Why does the tongue muscle feel so soft in an outspoken person? Because they're not holding in what they want to say, or stifling how they want to express themselves. They just do it. What comes out is sometimes positive. Other times it's negative. What I want to teach you by Volume 3 of this text is how to communicate in a way that is always received well, and that results in outcomes that are energetically positive for all parties involved.

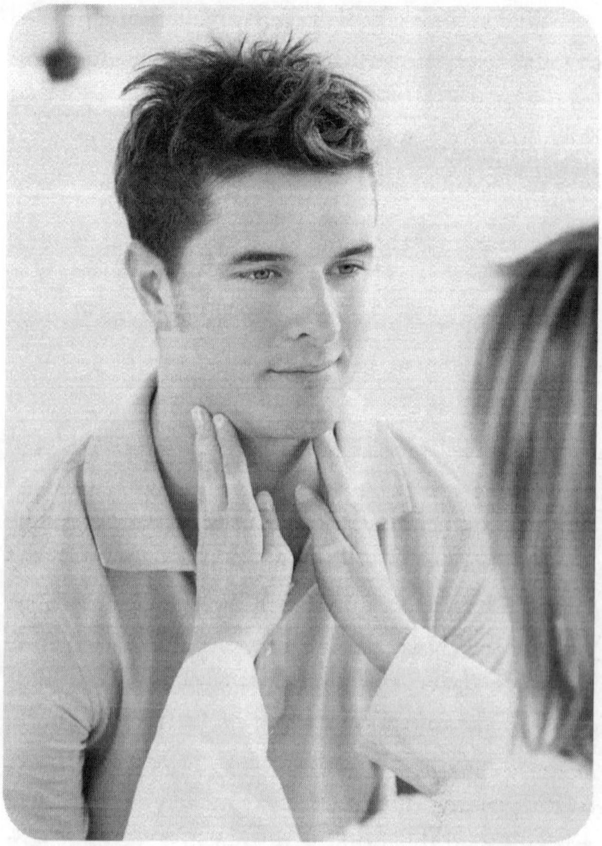

Figure 3.4

WHAT ARE THE EFFECTS OF A STRESSOR?

Emotional Charge is typically the result of energy draining emotions that have either gone unexpressed or have not resulted in satisfying outcome. Because the feeling still lives within the psyche, it is replayed through the limbic centers of the Brain, causing shifts in the Autonomic Nervous System and often leading to a pre-charged activation of the body's Fight-Or-Flight Nervous System.

In Fight-Or-Flight mode, the body will tend to stay on high alert for potential danger and tense muscles in anticipation of action. Also in anticipation of action, your body will overstimulate the release of a very precious stress-response hormone called Cortisol. Cortisol—from a hormonal perspective—is our life-force. In abundance, we feel vibrant. But with a deficiency, we often feel depleted and depressed.

Like all stressors, Emotional Charge creates an acidic environment within the body that leads to damage of the organs most associated with the Energy-Draining Reactions. Of course, this occurs at the cellular level and will initiate at least five of the seven-step healing response—Pain, Inflammation, Migration, Proliferation, and Scar Tissue. (Because most diets are deficient in alkalizing nutrients, Scar Tissue is often not broken down and the tissue is never completely remodeled.)

HOW DO WE RELEASE EMOTIONAL CHARGE?

Expression! Emotional Charge is dissipated from the Nervous System through expression. Pre-charging memories along the dendrites are released through the application of detailed healing plans including Primary Therapies, Complementary Therapies, Fine-Tuning Therapies, and Essential Therapies as detailed in chapter 2.

The basic idea is to express yourself to your level of satisfaction in constructive ways that include vocal expression and movement. Honor your first thought. Trust it. Believe in it. Act Upon it in constructive ways that utilize Energy-Cultivating Emotional Responses.

If your first thought regularly proves to be self-destructive, that is okay. It means that your heart has been significantly hurt, and that there is much to heal before you can use it as the resource for decision-making that it is designed to be. In these instances, it is appropriate to begin working with someone who can guide you in how to heal the pain in your heart. It's very important to begin working with people who've been there, and who have figured out how to grow stronger from the experience. Work with someone who knows how to take a negative heart-wrenching experience and turn it into a source of strength. These are the folks to work with. As you learn to transform negative energy into positive energy, your heart will start speaking more clearly in energy cultivating ways through the intuition of your first thought. As a result, when you call on your heart to help you make decisions, you will give yourself the opportunity to realize your dreams.

Acidic Cellular Environments— The Precursor to Fatigue

WHAT IS IT? Your body is designed to work within very specific and very narrow pH ranges. The pH of anything is classically defined by the amount of hydrogen in a substance, and is recorded on a logarithmic scale of 0 to 14. Substances at 7.0—like water—are said to be neutral. Substances between 0 and 6.99 are considered acidic. And substances between 7.01 and 14 are said to be alkaline (See **Figure 3.5**). What's interesting is that energy production thrives in a slightly alkaline pH of approximately 7.5. What's also interesting is that virtually every pH of your body is based upon the pH of your bloodstream, which is held under tight alkaline control of 7.35 to 7.45. If the pH of the blood falls below 7.35, then the pH within the cells will fall below the optimal 7.2. As the pH within the cell falls below 7.2, the cell takes on a relatively more acidic state. Acid leads to damage of the Mitochondria. And damage of the Mitochondria leads to interruptions in energy production, commonly experienced as fatigue.

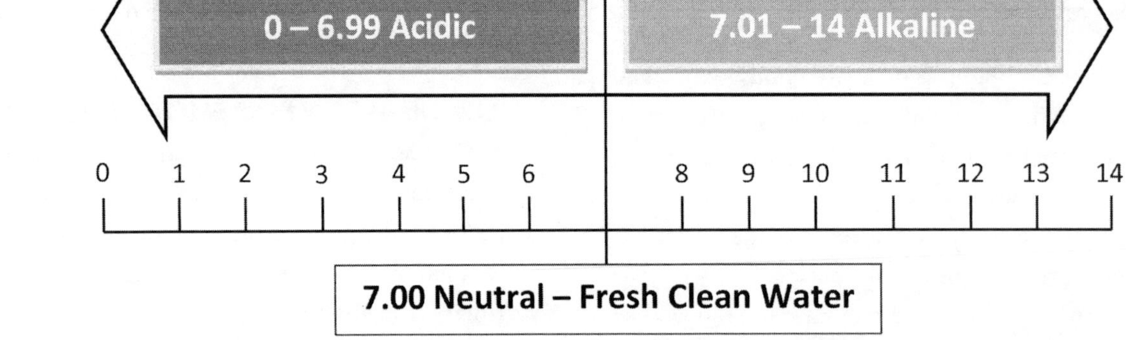

Figure 3.5
Understand that alkalinity is associated with energy production and optimal enzyme production, while acidity is associated with healthy immune function. However, when a tissue shifts away from its optimal state problems ensue. Tissues normally alkaline can become acidic while tissues normally acidic can become alkaline. From here energy and enzyme production suffers.

Tissue	Optimal pH Range for Energy Production
Blood	7.35 to 7.45
Extracellular Fluid	7.4
Intercellular Fluid (Cytosol)	7.2 to 7.45
Mitochondria—Within Cell	7.5
Smooth Endoplasmic Reticulum—Within Cell	7.2
Lymphatic Fluid	7.1 to 7.3
Cerebrospinal Fluid	7.3 or Higher
Small Intestine	7.0 to 8.0
Semen	7.2 to 8.0

Figure 3.6A
Optimal pH ranges for regions of the body associated with energy production.

While the aspects of the body associated with energy production enjoy a slightly alkaline pH, many parts of the body associated with immune function naturally maintain a slightly acidic pH (See **Figure 3.6B**). Acid pH also can create damage and what better to cause damage to the body than infections and environmental pollution? However, remember that even these pH levels are based on the alkaline pH of the bloodstream. Any shifts in blood pH toward a more acidic state can cause acidic pH levels of the Immune System to become more alkaline, and as a result, less effective.

Tissue	Optimal pH Range for Immune Function
Stomach Acid	1.2 to 2.0
Lysosomes—Within Cell	4.0 to 4.5
Hydrogen Peroxide—Within Neutrophils	5.5
Skin	4.2 to 5.6
Sweat	4.3 to 4.7
Tears	6.5
Saliva	6.0 to 6.8
Urine	6.0 to 6.8
Large Intestine	5.5 to 6.5
Vaginal Mucosa	3.8 to 4.5

Figure 3.6B
Optimal pH ranges for regions of the body associated with immune function.

When we consider Acidic Cellular Environments as stressors, we are focusing on the effect that pH has over two very important aspects of the body—the bloodstream, and the inside of the cell (intercellular fluid, Mitochondria, and the Smooth Endoplasmic Reticulum). Anything that causes these pH levels to shift into a state of acidity is a consideration for healing, because acid leads to damage. Damage to the Mitochondria—where ATP energy is produced—is the condition that creates fatigue, and ultimately, that leads to disease.

HOW IS IT CREATED?

Acidic Cellular Environments are created by any of the 4 Considerations for Healing, including Emotional Charge, Biomechanical Misalignments, and Scar Tissue. Acidic Cellular Environments also are created by nutrient deficiencies, industrialized fast-food diets, delayed food allergies, sedentary lifestyles, exposure to environmental pollution, constipation, congested Livers and Kidneys, and infections. From what you think to what you say, and especially to what you eat—anything that does not help promote your production of energy can lead to Acidic Cellular Environments. (See **Figure 3.7** on the next page)

WHAT ARE THE EFFECTS OF A STRESSOR?

Again, Acidic Cellular Environments lead to a classic cycle of damage. With damage occurring at the Mitochondrial level, ATP energy production is interrupted. Fatigue ensues, and the body shifts from an energy-producing powerhouse to a Bio-accumulating Organism. The body also will have to initiate a proactive healing response as a result of the damage. What we have not yet covered is information about pain signals, Inflammation, Migration, Proliferation, Maturation of Scar Tissue, and how these processes require a tremendous amount of energy. *So not only has the ability to produce energy been hampered, but the need for energy has increased.* If you are entering into this process of damage and repair all day long, every single day—because your diet is acidic or because your emotional states are reactionary and energy draining—then you will always be working from an energy deficit, and a state of fatigue. What comes next? Disease.

HOW DO WE ALLEVIATE ACIDIC CELLULAR ENVIRONMENTS?

First and foremost, use the Cycle of Influencing Energy® to your advantage by creating multiple points of entry into a healing cycle. In the next two chapters, you will learn what the Mitochondria of your cells need to produce energy. You also will learn what Eating Healthy really means. By Eating Healthy, you give your Mitochondria everything they need to produce energy, and as a result, energy is likely to be produced.

Additionally, consider the power of going Organic. Organic foods are a great way to support alkalinity in your bloodstream and inside your cells. Organic foods are superior to conventional foods because they have a higher nutrient density, a higher antioxidant potential, a higher enzyme capacity, a higher energy potential, and they are typically farmed in humane and sustainable ways. What's more, you get all of this without environmental pollution and bacterial infections. Every dollar spent on Organic foods is a vote cast for your future. When you choose Organic foods, you choose life.

If you follow the principles of Advanced Natural Medicine throughout this text, you will have more energy. Cultivating energy is as much about what you choose not to do, as what you choose to do. There isn't a doubt in my mind. I've seen it happen for thousands of people. I am a living proof of it, and I want you to be living proof of it as well.

Biomechanical Misalignments—How Your Posture Affects Your Breathing

WHAT ARE THEY? Kyphosis. Lordosis. Torsion. Scoliosis. Biomechanical Misalignments are body postures that restrict the body's ability to breathe effortlessly from the diaphragm. The importance of breath cannot be understated because Biomechanical Misalignments lead to a deficiency in oxygen. A body that is deficient in oxygen forces the Heart to pump faster and the Lungs to breathe faster. A body deficient in oxygen also speeds up and accumulates carbon dioxide, a very acidic substance that promotes stressful Acidic Cellular Environments. It's important to note that of all the substances available for nutrient consumption, oxygen is the most alkalizing. Therefore, a body that is misaligned physically experiences at least two major stressors—restriction of the diaphragm, which leads to the aforementioned acceleration of the Heart, Lungs and thought processes; and the development of stressful Acidic Cellular Environments.

Additionally, Biomechanical Misalignments force muscles to work harder than they need to, which leads to inefficiencies in movement and a waste of the very ATP essential for muscle contraction. Let me give you two examples to help illustrate my point.

First, I want you to take your arms and fold them across your chest as if you were hugging yourself. Next, lean forward and attempt to take the biggest breath that you can take. Was your breath labored and restricted from this exaggerated misalignment? Yes? Let's continue on.

As a comparison, I want you to sit back in your chair, but sit up as straight as possible with your hands—palms up—comfortably resting on your lap. Now, take the biggest breath you can take. Which one was bigger—the first or the second? Obviously, the second breath—while your body was more optimally aligned was more efficient. What's neat is that when your body is aligned, you also are able to conserve more energy in your muscles. You might be thinking that these are extreme postures? Well, they're not so extreme if you observe common body postures complete with sunken Hearts, slumped shoulders, and upper torsos leaning forward. Add to these body posture problems a Biomechanical Misalignment that can come from wearing a purse or a backpack, holding a baby, playing a musical instrument, swinging a golf club, or wearing a heavy tool belt. If you consider all the things we ask our bodies to do, it's not difficult to see how poor postures can create additional issues. Out of alignment, the breath becomes compromised and labored. This results in the accumulation of carbon dioxide, acidity, cellular damage, and fatigue. Your body is designed to work in an optimally aligned posture, and anything less doesn't feel very good. Poor posture can lead to stiff backs and necks with cricks in them.

As a second example, let's explore how misalignments actually waste energy. In order for a muscle to contract, it must have the energy necessary to facilitate the contraction of the muscle. When a body is misaligned, it compensates by recruiting additional muscles to accomplish the desired movement—even if that movement is simply standing up. *Therefore, a body that is misaligned uses more energy to perform a given action than a body that is optimally aligned. It takes more energy to live in a poor posture than it does in an optimally aligned posture.* For the second example, you will need to be standing.

One of the most common Biomechanical Misalignments is known as *forward* lean. Forward lean is similar to how a ski jumper leans into a jump while flying through the air. While this may be good for the ski jumper, it's not ideal for the rest of us. While standing, place your fingertips on the muscles that are located along the small of your back, closest to the spine (See **Figure 3.8**). Like a ski jumper, lean your entire body forward. Do you feel the muscles of your lower back tightening as they work harder to keep you upright? Can you feel your lower back muscles getting tighter? Can you feel any other muscles called into service?

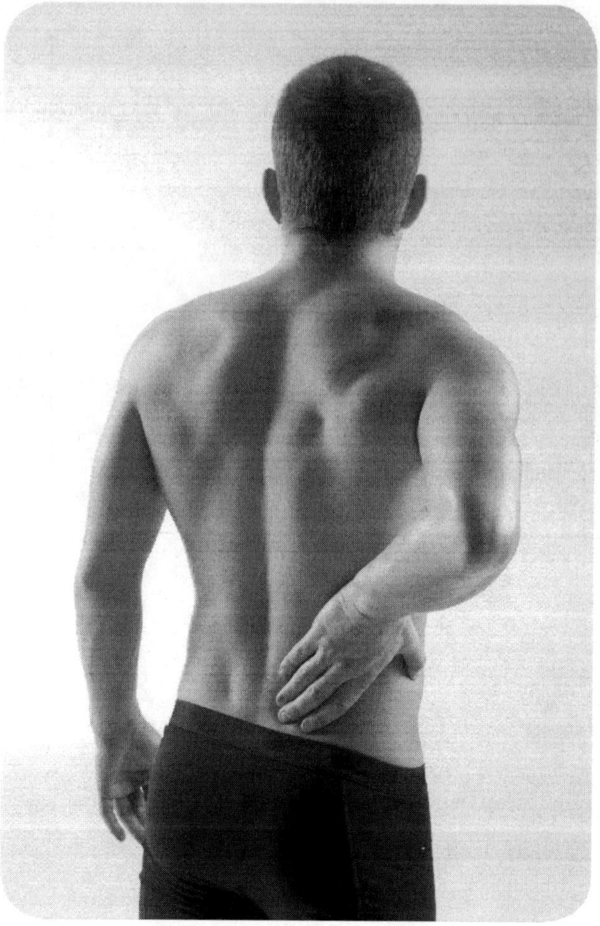

Figure 3.8

Figure 3.7

Alkalizing vs. Acidifying Foods and Lifestyle

(+4) Most Alkalizing	(+3) More Alkalizing	(+2) Alkalizing	(+1) Least Alkalizing	Category
Loving, Satisfied, Joyful, Enthusiastic, Authentic	Patient, Peaceful, Confident, Truthful, Encouraging	Trusting, Faithful, Passionate, Calm	Rational, Tolerant	**Perspectives/ Emotional State**
Active 5X/Week	Active 4X/Week	Active 3X/Week	Active 2X/Week	**Exercise**
Eat at Home with Family 5X per week	Eat at Home with Family 4x per week	Eat at Home with Family 3x per week	Eat at Home with Family 1 – 2x per week	**Lifestyle**
8+ Hours Uninterrupted	8 Hours Uninterrupted	7.5 Hours Uninterrupted	7 Hours Uninterrupted	**Sleep**
Breathing Practice 60+ min/day	Breathing Practice 45 min/day	Breathing Practice 30 min/day	Breathing Practice 15 min/day	**Blood Gases**
Cloves, Cinnamon Oregano, Basil Turmeric Parsley	Thyme Cumin	Green Tea Ginger Peppermint, Spearmint Marjoram	Curry Sage Licorice Root Burdock Root	**Herbs**
Avocado Persimmon Papayas Lemons, Limes Blueberries	Plums BlackBerries Oranges, Tangelos Mango Grapes with Seeds	Apple, Pear Pineapple Raspberries Strawberries Peach Kiwi	Apricot, Nectarine Honeydew, Cantaloupe Banana Currant, Cherries Cooked Tomatoes Watermelon	**Fruits**
Spinach, Kale, Collards Swiss Chard, Greens Broccoli, Arugula Nori, Wakame, Kombu Hijiki	Cucumber, Zucchini Parsnip Green Leaf, Romaine Brussels Sprouts Boy Choy Fermented Soy	Sweet Potato Beets, Cauliflower Carrots Bell Peppers Pumpkin & Squash Garlic, Onions	Soy Beans, Tofu Jicama, Celery Green Peas, Asparagus Adzuki Beans, Black Beans Kidney Beans, Green Beans Hummus	**Vegetables & Legumes**
Wheat Grass Chlorella, Spirulina Blue - Green Algae Miso Soup	Most Vegetable Based Soups	Oats Sumac Sorghum Lentils	Quinoa Millet Amaranth	**Grains, Cereals, Grass, Soups**
Sprouts	Walnuts Pecans	Almonds Pistachio Hazelnut	Pumpkin Seeds Brazil Nuts Shitake	**Sprouts, Nuts, Mushrooms & Seeds**
	Cod Liver Oil	Evening Primrose Oil Borage Oil Cold Pressed Extra Virgin Olive Oil Flax Seed Oil	Avocado Oil Coconut Oil	**Oils**
			Perhaps Sushi If it is Wild Caught	**Meat Fowl Wild Game Shellfish**
	Breast Milk	Oat Milk Hemp Milk Almond Milk	Coconut Milk Rice Milk Soy Milk	**Dairy & Alternative Milks**
Herbal Organic Teas Ginseng Bicarbonate	High Quality Waters* Mineral Water	Sake with Miso Espresso Coffee	Filtered Water Honey Wine Red Wine	**Beverages**
Sea Salt		Black Strap Molasses Apple Cider Vinegar Umeboshi Stevia	Maple Syrup Raw Honey Raw Agave Rice Syrup	**Sweeteners Seasonings**
		Broad Spectrum Probiotics	Multivitamins, Antioxidants	**Extra**
				Totals

Reference 1. Prior, Wu. 'Oxygen Radical Absorbance Capacity of Selected Foods- 2007'. (Based on 20 References) 2. Mateljan. 'The World's Healthiest Foods' 2007. (based on 150+ References)

Category	(-1) Least Acidifying	(-2) Acidifying	(-3) More Acidifying	(-4) Most Acidifying
Perspectives/ Emotional State	Indifferent, Indecisive	Distrustful, Afraid, Lonely, Doubtful	Angry, Complaining, Frustrated, Isolated	Judgmental, Repressed, Controlling
Exercise	Active Without Sweating	Sedentary	Sedentary With Fast Food Diet	Sedentary + Fast Food + Sugar/Alcohol
Lifestyle	Eat Fast Food 1 – 2x per week	Eat Fast Food 3x per week	Eat Fast Food 4x per week	Eat Fast Food 5x per week
Sleep	6 Hours Uninterrupted	6 - 7 Hours Interrupted	5-6 Hours Interrupted	Less Than 5 Hours Total
Blood Gases	Shallow Breather	Shallow Breather w/ Kyphosis	Snore While Sleeping	Diagnosed with Sleep Apnea
Herbs				
Fruits	Sour Cherries Rhubarb Prune Raisin Dates	Cranberries Raw Tomatoes	Canned Fruit Shelf Juices w/ Sugar/Corn Syrup	All Non-Organic Fruit
Vegetables & Legumes	Potatoes String Beans Chick Peas **Note: When Presoaked, Sprouted Beans Become More Alkalizing – Dr. Michio Kushi**	White Beans Navy Beans Pinto Beans	Processed Soy Products	All Non-Organic Vegetables
Grains, Cereals, Grass, Soups	Brown Rice Kasha Teff	Buckwheat Wheat Semolina Farina Spelt	Maize Corn Rye Barley White Rice	White Bread
Sprouts, Nuts, Mushrooms & Seeds	Peanuts Pine nuts Sunflower Seeds	Cashews		
Oils	Sesame Oil Grape Seed Oil Sunflower Oil Almond Oil Peanut Oil	Safflower Oil		Fried Foods Trans Fatty Acids Partially Hydrogenated Oils Crisco
Meat Fowl Wild Game Shellfish	**All Organic Free Range Meats & Eggs** **Pacific Wild Caught Fish**	Goat, Lamb Goose Turkey Shrimp Duck, Venison	Chicken Beef Eggs Crab, Scallops	Pork Oysters Lobsters Cat Fish Atlantic/Farmed Fish
Dairy & Alternative Milks	Goat cheese Sheep cheese Yogurt Goat Products	Aged Cheese Organic Dairy Products	Casein	Cheese Cow Milk Ice Cream Pus Cells
Beverages	Black Tea Sake	Lipton Tea	I Drink___Cups of Coffee per day	I Drink___Sodas, Diet Sodas, Alcoholic Beverages per day
Sweeteners Seasonings	Processed Honey Raw Sugar Brown Sugar	Vanilla	White Sugar Jams/Jellies Yeast	NutraSweet Equal Sweet n Low Splenda High Fructose Corn Syrup
Extra	L. Acidophilus			Antibiotics
Totals				

As a comparison, let's demonstrate how optimal alignment begins in the feet, and how easy it is to create in your body. Activate your feet by lifting your toes up, and spreading them apart. Do you notice how your body weight naturally rocks back, and how it becomes distributed through your heal? At this point, your legs, pelvis, and upper torso are aligned, while the balls of your feet are used for additional balance. Notice how your spine begins to lengthen upward?

Feel your lower back muscles again, and make note of how much softer they feel in this posture. Your body is no longer overworking just to stand up. Because you are optimally aligned, your spine has lengthened, and as a result, your rib cage moves more freely during respiration. A bigger breath leads to more oxygen, more alkalinity, and greater energy production. Your body is now beginning to maximize the efficiency of its design.

As a final comparison, allow your feet to relax. Take notice of how your body begins to lean forward again. Feel your back muscles tighten, and then activate your feet again to compare the difference between what it feels like to be Biomechanically Misaligned with how it feels when you are optimally aligned.

Understand the simplicity of this concept. By activating your feet consistently throughout the day, you consistently return your entire body to optimal alignment and create space along your spinal column. Is this something you can do while standing in your shoes? Yes. Is this something you can do while walking? Yes. Is this something you can even do while sitting down? Yes. Activating your toes trains your body to reflexively lift throughout the entire spinal column—even while sitting. This routine and inexpensive practice of Advanced Natural Medicine is perfect for anyone who routinely suffers from back or neck problems. More space, more movement, more energy—through conservation.

WHAT CREATES THEM?

When you think of Biomechanical Misalignments and what causes them, a person's inattentiveness to posture is a major contributing factor. This is something I'm sure we can all relate to. Utilizing the Cycle of Influencing Energy®, recall that emotion influences the Anatomy of our posture. Drawing from this concept, it is safe to reason that emotion plays a HUGE role in Biomechanical Misalignments. Similarly, as will be exemplified in the following subchapter, Scar Tissue from previous injuries and surgeries also can play a significant role in Biomechanical Misalignments. If you are beginning to see that every stress can create a snowball effect for your body, then you are beginning to understand this thought process. But let's delve a little deeper into Biomechanical Misalignments.

What force is constantly pulling down on your body? If you guessed gravity, then you are correct. Gravity is constantly pulling you down, but alignment provides a wonderful solution. Optimal alignment gives you the ability to function within the earth's gravitational pull, with the least amount of energy expended. This prevents fatigue. It is because of gravity that we say our posture begins from the feet up, as demonstrated in our previous example. I have included a chart of common misalignments that is divided into seven anatomical regions unique to Release Point Therapy® (See **Figure 3.9** on the next page). I will not detail or analyze various postures at this time, as these will be addressed in future texts.

WHAT ARE THE EFFECTS OF A STRESSOR?

With Biomechanical Misalignments, breathing becomes more difficult. As a result, breathing and heart rates speed up, and the body shifts into a protective Fight-Or-Flight state to meet the cellular demand for oxygen. Just by how our bodies stand and sit—how we hold ourselves—changes how our Nervous System functions. How we hold our bodies changes how we breathe, how frequently we breathe, and even how we think. When your body perceives a deficiency in oxygen, it speeds up due to the accumulation of carbon dioxide, which creates Acidic Cellular Environments. Your body is designed to continue and sustain life—this is your body's basic, pre-wired logic. If your cells are getting enough oxygen, your body is able to relax. If your cells are not getting enough oxygen, then everything

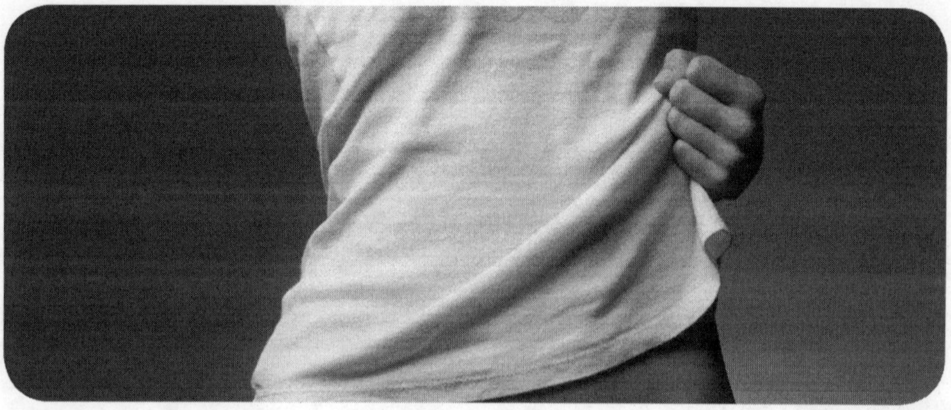

Figure 3.10

speeds up. It all revolves around oxygen—your body has to deliver oxygen to your cells. Oxygen leads to alkalinity and the production of energy; lack of oxygen leads to fatigue, and ultimately, to disease.

HOW DO WE ALLEVIATE BIOMECHANICAL MISALIGNMENTS?

Posture begins from the ground up. Make sure that your shoes allow you to utilize all of your foot muscles. Too often, we wear shoes that are too small for the foot. This causes individual foot muscles to atrophy. A person who walks barefoot is typically more concerned about stepping on something painful, and as a result, activates his or her feel more frequently. A person who lives life in his or her shoes has a tendency to let the feet fall asleep. Athletic practice without shoes is another advantage of practicing Yoga—it gives participants an opportunity to activate their feet throughout the entire practice.

Additionally, if you happen to favor one side of your body—as when you're holding your kids on your hip, or playing sports or a musical instrument—be sure to occasionally place the kids on the other hip or swing from the other side. Balance your body out. It doesn't necessarily take equal repetitions from the other side of your body to create balance—only the attention necessary to do it more than occasionally.

Still, if you're playing a musical instrument and you aren't able to play it from the other side, remember that this is what Yoga is all about. Yoga is about creating muscular and skeletal balance throughout the body. A Yoga asana or posture practice helps create optimal alignment while also teaching you how to breath efficiently. Yoga is medicine that's been around for thousands of years. It also is no accident that Yoga has a growing number of practitioners—more than any other healing modality today.

Scar Tissue—Principle of Advanced Natural Medicine #5:

WHAT IS IT? Scar Tissues—also known as myofascial adhesions—are weak collagen fibers formed by fibroblast cells that help reinforce previously injured tissue. A scar on the Skin is one form, but the type of Scar Tissue we are discussing occurs within the muscles and soft tissues of the body.

Let's illustrate the effects of Scar Tissue with a quick example. If you take a corner of your shirt and fold it over at the shoulder three times, you will begin to feel the shirt tightening around your shoulder joint. This is precisely the effect that Scar Tissue has on the body. It makes the body tighter than it needs to be. If you twist the folded corner of your shirt just a little bit more, you'll notice lines of tension starting to form (See **Figure 3.10**). In a similar way, these lines of tension that are transmitted throughout your body allow Scar Tissue to create Biomechanical Misalignments. If you attempt to raise your arm

Figure 3.9

Release Point Therapy ~ Anatomical Levels Assessments and Release Points

Anatomical Level	*Location*	*Important Structural Muscles*	*Visual Assessment*
7	Clavicles to top of the Head	Scalenes, Levator Scapulae, Splenius, SCM Masseter` Temporalis` Lateral Pterygoid` Medial Pterygoid` Rectus Capitis Posterior", Obliquus Capitis Inferior", Obliquus Capitis Superior	***Forward Head Carriage:*** Reveals chronic tension in the Scalenes, Levator Scapulae, Splenius and Lower ALs. ***Unlevel & Rotated Eye Sockets:*** indicates that Sphenoid Bone is misaligned and cranial rhythms are that disrupted.
6	Xiphoid Process to Clavicles	Pectoralis Maj&Min, Rhomboids, Serratus Anterior, Supraspinatus^^ Infraspinatus^^ Teres Minor^^ Subscapularis^^	***Kyphosis, Hood of the Cobra:*** Reveals a withdrawn heart and tension in the Pericardium typically consistent with scarring between the Diaphragm and Sternum. ***Pectoralis Minors Atrophy in a Contracted State***. ***Scoliosis & Spinal Torsion:*** Indicates imbalanced muscles from left to right sides of the body.
5	12th Ribs to Xiphoid Process	Diaphragm	***Elevated Collar Bones:*** Indicates that the person is using the Scalenes as an accessory respiration muscle transmitting tension to the Levator Scapula. ***Absent Xiphoid Process:*** On Palpation the XP can be tucked underneath the sternum due to ***Diaphragm Atrophying in a Contracted State***.
4	Iliac Crests to 12th Ribs	Psoas^ Quadratus Lumborum^ Erector Spinae	***Lordosis:*** Always indicates tension in the Psoas and neighboring QLs and Erector Spinae. ***In fact, EVERY spinal misalignment involves Psoas Tension.***
3	Ischial Tuberosities to Iliac Crests	Piriformis** Superior Gemellus** Obturator Internus** Inferior Gemellus** Quadratus Femoris**, Iliacus, TFL, Gluteus Maximus	***Laterally Rotated Feet*** indicates tension in the Piriformis Muscle & Lateral (Posterior) Rotators that can lead to Sciatica. ***Tight Hips:*** Narrow hips, short shuffling gait.
2	Knees to Ischial Tuberosities	Semitendonsous* Semimembranosus* Biceps Femoris* Rectus Femoris, Vastus Medialis, IT Band, Adductor Magnus	***Forward Lean of the Body:*** Indicates Contracted Hamstrings and often times Erector Spinae and Psoas. ***Hamstrings can and will atrophy in a contracted state due to seated lifestyles.*** ***Tight Rope Walking:*** Indicates Tight & Emotionally Charged Adductors. ***Short/Shuffling Gait:*** Typically denotes contracted Rectus Femoris, TFL, and Gluteus Maximus.
1	Soles of the Feet to Knees	Peroneus Longus Tibialis Anterior Gastrocnemeus Soleus Flexor Digitorum Longus Extensor Digitorum Longus	***Flat Feet:*** Indicates that the Peroneus Longus is typically atrophied. Likely a result of scar tissue adhering it to the neighboring Soleus. ***Knocked Knees:*** Indicates Flat Feet and Structural Shortening of the IT Band.

Muscle Groups - * denotes Hamstrings, ** denotes Posterior Lateral Rotators, ^ denotes Posterior Abdominal Wall, ^^ denotes Rotator Cuff, ` denotes Muscles of Mastication, "denotes Suboccipital Triangle

Myofascial Meridian Releases - AL3 ~ Piriformis, AL4 ~ Quadratus Lumborum and Psoas, AL5 ~ Diaphragm, AL6 ~ Pectoralis Minor and Rotator Cuff, AL7 ~ Scalene, TMJ, and Occiput

Rationale	*Major Release Points*
Scalenes, Levators and Splenius in tension, will transmit tension to the Suboccipital Muscles and ultimately impair nerve flow through the Brachial Plexus, Suboccipital Nerve as well as restrict blood flow through the Vertebral Artery to the Brain. Muscles of Mastication when overly toned will disrupt the alignments and rhythms of Cranial bones. Biomechanical Misalignments in the cranium and jaw from excessive thought as well as kyphotic postures will greatly contribute to pain from Carpal Tunnel Syndrome and vice versa. Always treat the neck to heal shoulder, elbow, wrist and hand pain.	Suboccipital triangle at **Gall Bladder 20** . The Gate of Heaven at **Governing Vessel 16** . Third Eye at **Ying Tang** . Masseter along the **Gall Bladder Meridian** . Scalenes at **Small Intestine 16.** Muscles of Mastication at **Stomach 3 thru 8, Small Intestine 17 thru 19, & Gall Bladder 2**. Levator Scapulae at **Small Intestine 13** .
A contracted Pec Minor will restrict the rib cage's ability to expand during inspiration thereby over stimulating the 'Fight or Flight' Sympathetic Nervous System and cause the body to use accessory muscles for inspiration thus quickening the breath and heart rates. Scoliosis often causes the rib cage to ossify misshapen which can lead to a lifetime of chronic back pain.	Insertion of the Pec Minor at **Lung 1 & 2** . Insertion of Pec Major at Humoral Head. Medial Border of the Scapula for Rhomboids, Subscapularis, and Serratus Anterior. Rotator Cuff Muscles at **Triple Heater 14, Small Intestine 9 thru 12** . Medial Epicondyle of the Humerus and along **Heart Meridian** . Lateral Epicondyle of the Humerus and along the **Large Intestine Meridian** .
Without sufficient Diaphragm tone and Mobility, Autonomic Balance, Respiration, Spinal Mobilization, and Digestion become impaired as organs become stagnant with accumulated toxic deposits.	Xiphoid Process at **Conception Vessel 12** . Anterior Diaphragmatic Release Points along the inferior border of the rib cage.
Because of their proximity to the organs of digestion these muscles are prone to collecting excess metabolic acidity from diet and digestion. This leaves them susceptible to injury from inflammation created by Acidic Blood & Tissue pH.	***Lateral Border of the Erector Spinae just inferior to the 12th Rib at Gall Bladder 25.*** Thoracolumbar Fascia. Origin of the Quadratus Lumborum at the Iliac Crest.
Tension in Posterior Rotators will shift the Pelvis forward and tilt it anteriorly downward. The result is typically a Lordodic spinal alignment. The Piriformis can also act to lock the Sacrum, thus dampening flow of Kundalini energy through the Chakras and contributing greatly to the development of Sciatica.	Origin of the Erector Spinae and Gluteus Maximus at the **Sacrum & Sacroilliac Joint**. Midpoint of the Piriformis at **Gall Bladder 30.**
Hamstrings attach directly to Ischial Tuberosity of Pelvis and can therefore disrupt the alignment of the Pelvis when in Chronic Tension resulting from sitting for prolonged periods of time each day for years. Similarly, the Rectus Femoris will atrophy due to lack of use and thus offer little assistance to the Iliopsoas.	IT Band along the **Gall Bladder Meridian.** Origin of the Rectus Femoris at **Stomach 31** . Myofascial channels along the Rectus Femoris consistent with the **Stomach and Spleen-Pancreas Meridians.** Ischial Tuberosities at **Urinary Bladder 36.** Insertion of the Illio-Psoas at the Lesser Trochanter - this point also effectively releases the Adductor Magnus and Semimembranosis/Semitendonosis.
Peroneus Longus & Tibialis Anterior tendons form the Transverse Arch of the Foot. Flat Feet lead to an internal rotation of the ankles that cause the knees to 'knock' inward and chronically shorten the IT Bands. As a result the hips commonly rotate anteriorly downward leading to a lordodic posture and compression of the spinal column.	Base of 1st Metatarsal and Medial Cuneiform at **Kidney 1 & 2**. Tendon of the Peroneus Longus behind the 5th Metatarsal at **Urinary Bladder 62, 63, & 64. Origin of the Peroneus Longus on the Head of the Fibula at Gall Bladder 34** , Origin of the Tibialis Anterior at **Stomach 36** . Achiles Tendon at **Kidney 3 and Urinary Bladder 60**. Dorsal Surface of the Food and Ankle.

while holding the twisted fold of your shirt, you'll notice that it is difficult to raise your arm. Scar Tissue consumes space, thereby restricting motion and the flow of energy.

Scar Tissue can be found wherever there is fascia—this includes Muscles, Tendons, Ligaments, areas around bones and in each and every organ. Fascia is your body's most abundant connective tissue, and it runs continuously from just beneath your Skin, all the way to your bones, and from the bottom of your feet, to the top of your head. Fascia surrounds and penetrates every muscle and organ of your body, acting as a carrier tissue for nerves, blood vessels, and lymphatic chains.

WHAT CREATES IT?

Any source of damage—be it Emotional Charge, Acidic Cellular Environments, Biomechanical Misalignments, and even existing Scar Tissue—can create more Scar Tissue. Your body is responsible for healing any and all damage, and Scar Tissue is an end point for all injuries. Ultimately, what we have to understand is that *any stress leads to Acidic Cellular Environments; Acidic Cellular Environments lead to damage; and damage always leads to the formation of Scar Tissue (Principle of Advanced Natural Medicine #5).* So if Scar Tissue accumulates more readily than enzymes can break it down, then a part of the body's natural Healing Process can become part of the problem.

WHAT ARE THE EFFECTS OF A STRESSOR?

Scar Tissue blocks the flow of energy through internal and surface meridian energy pathways, which are covered in chapter 6. For now, imagine that a meridian energy pathway is just like a river. Imagine you're standing next to a river, and you're seeing water trickling along slowly. You look upstream and see a beaver dam, which is built with loose pieces of wood and debris, blocking the flow of the river. The water in the river is akin to the energy flow within your meridian energy pathways. Similarly, the actual dam is akin to Scar Tissue accumulation restricting the flow. Water pools in front of the dam, while water downstream flows weak and slow. Scar Tissue restricts the flow of energy, just as a dam restricts the flow of a river.

Scar Tissue disrupts the flow of energy through internal and surface meridian energy pathways, and it can remain in the body for a lifetime if it's not properly treated. Advanced Natural Medicine is what affords us the most sophisticated multilevel treatment for Scar Tissue, so that we are able to remove obstacles to cure.

Perhaps the words "energy" and "meridians" are too ambiguous for you right now. No worries. Let's revisit the first principle of Advanced Natural Medicine: Where there's space, there's movement. Where there's movement, there's energy. Where there's energy, disease cannot exist. Scar Tissue—just like the dam—consumes space. It also compressed four very vital tissues—nerves, arteries, veins, and lymph. In doing so, it creates a locally acidic cellular environment that leads to damage and the formation of more Scar Tissue. This is the recipe for an injury that never seems to heal, or for an injury that has prevented you from feeling normal since it occurred.

Should the body be able to effectively breakdown that Scar Tissue once your body has healed the tissue? Yes. But the reason most bodies don't effectively breakdown Scar Tissue is because most people don't move enough, and they don't eat enough alkalizing Organic, nutrient-dense foods. As a result, most bodies don't have the enzyme production needed to reabsorb Scar Tissue.

For many Healing Processes, a common misconception is that treating the Biochemistry will be enough. The truth is that natural healing often requires multiple points of energy to create a positive shift in health. If we can help create space, then movement and energy production will result. If we can get the blood cleaned and full of nutrients that are essential for energy production, then we've got a chance. If we can get the Scar Tissue out of your system, then your energy fields will reopen. If we can get this accomplished, inspire you to participate, and take control of your thoughts, responses, and life, then you are in the best possible position to heal. And guess what so often happens as a result of all this? Disease disappears.

HOW DO WE ALLEVIATE SCAR TISSUE?

Release Point Therapy, Sauna Therapy, and an alkaline bloodstream are the best ways to facilitate the removal of myofascial adhesions. By creating Alkaline Cellular Environments, we are able to help the body increase its own energy and enzyme production so that Scar Tissues—located deep within organs and places where hands can't reach—are broken down. A good massage becomes a GREAT massage when the body is alkaline. And a little sweating out of the toxins immediately after a massage also makes all the difference in the world.

LISTENING TO YOUR AMAZING BODY

In chapter 1, we asked, "What stresses you out?" We also helped you come up with a few stressors resulting from Emotional Charge. Now it's time for some fun. Let's develop a more thorough understanding of what stresses your body out. Answer the questions in each of the following categories to develop a better understanding of your own personal obstacles to cure that are draining your energy.

Emotional Charge

(Refer to the Genesis Five-Element Chart **Figure 2.2** for assistance)

When you are stressed out, what are your top three Energy-Draining Reactions, and which organs do they adversely affect?

	Energy-Draining Reaction	Yin Organ Affected	Yang Organ Affected
Ex.	*Frustration*	*Liver*	*Gallbladder*
1.			
2.			
3.			

Do any of these emotions create an acidic cellular environment? Yes No

(*Hint: The correct answer is Yes.*)

Acidic Cellular Environments

A 'Yes' answer to any of the following questions suggests an acidic cellular environment.

1. Is your diet less than 80 percent Organic?

   Yes No

2. Do you supplement your diet with nutrients and herbs less than three times a week?

   Yes No

3. Do you eat industrialized Fast-foods or frozen foods?

   Yes No

4. Do you drink at least one soda, energy drink, alcoholic beverage or coffee each day?

   Yes No

5. Do you eat foods that your Immune System has a delayed response to? (If you haven't been tested for delayed food allergies answer 'Yes')

   Yes No

6. Do you exercise less than thirty minutes three times per week?

   Yes No

7. Does your home have chemical cleaners, herbicides, and flooring?

   Yes No

8. Do you smoke?

   Yes No

9. Do you have silver amalgam fillings in your mouth?

   Yes No

10. Do you have less than one bowel movement per day?

    Yes No

11. Have you taken more than five to ten rounds of antibiotics in your life?

    Yes No

12. Are you currently taking pharmaceutical medicine for acid reflux?

    Yes No

13. Are you currently taking more than two pharmaceutical medications?

    Yes No

14. Do you use recreational drugs of any kind?

    Yes No

15. Do the whites of your eyes appear bloodshot?

    Yes No

16. Does your Skin regularly itch, burn, or appear red and inflamed?

    Yes No

17. Do your joints often ache or feel stiff?

    Yes No

Biomechanical Misalignments
(Refer to **Figure 3.9** for assistance)
A 'Yes' answer to any of the following questions suggests the presence of Biomechanical Misalignments.

1. Do you have flat feet?

   Yes No

2. Do your feet point in opposite directions when standing or walking?

   Yes No

3. Do you regularly wear high heels?

   Yes No

4. Do you regularly wear shoes that constrict your toes?

   Yes No

5. When walking and talking, do you happen to veer away or into the person you are talking to?

   Yes No

6. Do your footprints appear as if they are in one straight line?

   Yes No

7. Do you have a spinal misalignment such as a Lordosis, Scoliosis, or Kyphosis?

   Yes No

8. Do your shoulders slump?

   Yes No

9. Does your neck stick out and forward?

   Yes No

10. Does your body lean forward when standing?

    Yes No

11. Is your resting heart rate higher than seventy beats per minute?

    Yes No

12. Would you describe yourself as a shallow breather?

    Yes No

Scar Tissue

Beginning with your most recent injury, list every moderate to major injury you have experienced in your lifetime, including broken bones, Ligament tears, car accidents, sporting accidents, major falls, head injuries, and others.

	Year	Injury
1.		
2.		
3.		
4.		
5.		

Beginning with your most recent, list all previous surgeries.

	Year	Surgery
1.		
2.		
3.		
4.		
5.		

Find the tension, find the Scar Tissue. Where does your body routinely feel tense? List your top three locations (e.g. lower back, wrist, neck).

	Tension
1.	
2.	
3.	

Congratulations! You have just learned almost every way that your body experiences stress. As a result, you've also discovered the many ways that you lose energy every day. Now, let's do something about it.

What You Can Do To Cultivate Energy Today

Every single stress outlined in the 4 Considerations for Healing leads to the development of Acidic Cellular Environments and damage to your Mitochondrial Energy Production. In the next chapter, you will learn a great deal about Mitochondria and what they need to produce energy. For now, understand that producing energy has as much to do with avoiding stressors as it does with giving the body what it needs to produce energy.

For one week, you will select two stressors and practice the Alkalizing Healing Plan that follows to help create a more Alkaline Cellular Environment for optimal energy production. Take pictures of yourself and detail your moods the day before you begin, and do the same thing on day seven. What improvements did you experience?

RESOLUTION #4

Select two stressors to avoid for one week.

1.____

2.____

HEALING JOURNAL RECORDING

Record in your Healing Journal your moods, thoughts, and positive experiences throughout the week—both after your breathing practice and at the end of your workday. What improvements do you notice in your day?

Good Luck!

ALKALIZING HEALING PLAN

	Therapy	Instruction
Primary Therapy	Organic Clinical Nutrition	Eat something Organic, green, and rich in chlorophyll every day. Eat 80 percent or more Organic.
Complementary Therapy	Breathing Practice	Upon waking, and before starting your morning routine, breathe silently for fifteen to thirty minutes.
Complementary Therapy	Yoga	Activate your feet frequently throughout the day while standing, walking, or sitting.
Fine-Tuning Therapy	Meditation	At the conclusion of your breathing practice, think of anything that brings a smile to your face.
Essential Therapy	Laughter Before Bed	Read, watch, or listen to something that makes you laugh before you go to sleep for the night.

CHAPTER 4: THE MIGHTY MITOCHONDRIA

The Secret Ingredient to All Healing

Interesting insights to look for in this chapter:

- There's another organism living inside each of your cells.
- Eating something green for energy production and detoxification.
- 550,000,000,000,000,000,000 in the blink of an eye.
- Every essential nutrient for energy production.

Principle of Advanced Natural Medicine #6:

When the amount of stress in our bodies and in our lives exceeds our Mitochondrial ability to produce energy, fatigue can be the only possible outcome.

Populations of Powerhouses

Energy production and all life as we perceive it can be directly attributed to little cellular organelles known as Mitochondria (See **Figure 4.1**).

Did you know that your body is comprised of between fifty to seventy-five trillion cells (that's as many as 75,000,000,000,000—a whole lot of zeros right?). Within each and every cell are little powerhouses called Mitochondria. The number of Mitochondria per cell varies depending on the type of cell and the function it is designed for. The number of Mitochondria per cell will also vary based upon the availability of fuel (glucose and glucose derivatives), essential nutrients for energy production, and oxygen. Finally, the number of Mitochondria per cell will vary based on stress levels (as detailed by the 4 Considerations for Healing), your physical activity, and the genetic integrity of their individual DNA. That's right—the Mitochondria within your cells have their very own DNA. This means that at one point in our evolutionary history, they were not a part of us. What they found out—and what your body already knows—is that we work incredibly well together. We give them energy in the form they need, and they give us energy in the way that we need it—it's a wonderfully reciprocal relationship.

The relative population of Mitochondria per cell can range from as little as one to as many as several thousand per cell. Some researchers report that there are as many as ten thousand Mitochondria per cell in certain tissues. A typical cell will host between two hundred to four hundred Mitochondria, with major organs like the Liver, Heart, Muscles, and Kidneys hosting between one thousand to five thousand Mitochondria per cell. Thus, the more important the function, the greater the need for energy; and the greater the need for energy, the more Mitochondria per cell. For instance, it is estimated that Mitochondria make up approximately 20 percent of a Liver cell's total weight, and an even higher percentage of a Heart cell's total weight. The point is that your body—with the essential assistance of the Mitochondria—is designed to produced vast amounts of energy in the form of Adenosine 5' Triphosphate (ATP).

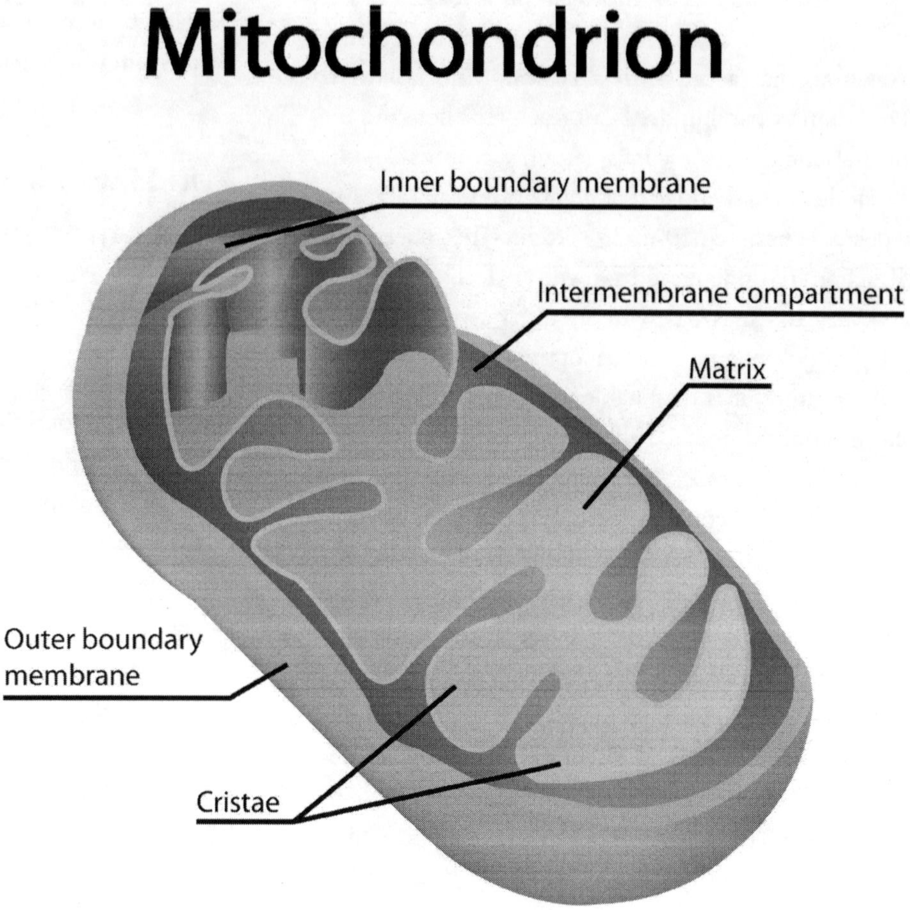

Figure 4.1
Final assembly of ATP takes place along the Inner Membrane.

In addition, your Mitochondria work together like a well-coordinated team. In fact, some researchers have started looking at Mitochondria in a unique way. Rather than taking interest in the relative populations per cell, they have begun to study total Mitochondrial mass per cell based on the Mitochondria's unique DNA signatures. This testing methodology allows researchers to more easily study relative changes due to age, environmental pollution, disease, nutrient depletion, and stress. These researchers have theorized that individual Mitochondria team up to form a single-branched structure within each cell that is dedicated to maximizing the production of ATP. Imagine ten thousand solar panel arrays branched together to power a single house—sounds like abundance of design to me!

A linear thought process might suggest that the Mitochondrial populations per cell remain relatively constant, independent of the variables life presents. This concept would be nice, but it is based more on fantasy than reality. While it may be unrealistic to assume that a cell with a typical Mitochondrial population of two hundred can reach ten thousand in optimal circumstances, it is certainly reasonable—if not modest—to theorize that populations can increase or decrease between 10 to 25 percent. The concept of Mitochondrial population growth or decline is not a new one, and it is based upon athletic performance and genetic potential. Under optimal circumstances while training, it is reasonable to assert that a person who has not yet reached their peak performance can improve their athletic performance by about 10 to 25 percent from where they first start. However, once their performance begins to peak, drastic gains in performance typically cannot be achieved naturally because Mitochondria will only grow to a certain population density in each cell. With this theory of Mitochondrial growth, a population of 200 could reach an Energetic peak of 250 or an Energetic valley of 150 per cell. Therefore, the cell reaching a population of 250 has entered into peak performance range, while the cell lagging with a population of 150 is indicative of fatigue, and possibly disease.

What I want you to take away from this chapter are some basics for Mitochondrial Energy Production, and how you can help your body produce optimal quantities of ATP every day. So how do you know when your Mitochondrial populations per cell are growing, versus when they are regressing? It's quite simple—look to your moods, or what we have referred to in the Cycle of Influencing Energy® as emotion.

If you are actively pursuing your dreams, then I can assure you that your Mitochondrial populations are growing. If you are consistently and effortlessly loving, happy, calm, truthful, patient, and confident, then I can guarantee that your Mitochondrial populations are growing, or that they have reached their peak. If you are practicing Energy-Cultivating Responses as detailed in **Figure 2.2**, then your Mitochondria are growing to their fullest cellular capacity and working as efficiently as the health of their DNA will permit.

Let's look at what kicks off this symbiotic relationship by looking at some of your body's most basic needs from the perspective of your Mitochondria.

You Have Needs... Your Mitochondria Have Needs Too

Mitochondria are quite intelligent. In fact, it is safe to say that they have their own consciousness as a result of having their own DNA. Much like us, they require a purpose to validate their production of energy. If the purpose is negativity, complaining, or vindictiveness—or any of the destructive Energy-Draining Reactions—then what incentive do Mitochondria have to produce energy? What is in it for them? Understand that your body was not designed for hatred, animosity, or negativity, which is why none of these feelings are enjoyable. You were designed in a much grander image. Think about this: What is more important than the pursuit of satisfaction, the pursuit of happiness, and the enjoyment of life? Joy is what our bodies live for, and this is what our bodies have been designed to experience. How do we know this? People who are happy live longer healthier lives.

Your body is designed to experience joy. If a person has no hope for the future—if they've given up on life—then their Mitochondria will give up on them. The Mitochondria have their own intelligence. They are engaged in a symbiotic relationship that depends on you. Thus, they will reciprocate what they are given. Without hope for the future, Mitochondria have no reason to continue because their job is to support the physical body so that the spirit living within can pursue its dreams. That's their job. So when there are no dreams to pursue, when there is no hope for the present or future, then Mitochondria think: "What am I doing here? You're wasting my time." Populations dwindle, and the #1 root cause of all disease—fatigue—becomes your reality.

Mitochondria simply will not function at their peak for prolonged periods of time without a purpose—they just won't do it. I have observed this over and over again in patients. I can give patients without dreams the best nutrients. They can be on the best exercise regimen. But if they are truly refusing to develop dreams, or if they are sabotaging themselves with negative internal dialogue, then their body will not produce energy. Any gains they realize will be very limited. Conversely, if a patient has goals and dreams that they want to achieve, then these are the people who have the best chance of healing. If I give the person who has a purpose in life the nutrients they need for energy production, then they get better. This turnaround can be quick and dramatic—like twenty-eight-days-later dramatic. The presence of dreams, a purpose, and some choice nutrients create Mitochondrial magic.

The point I want to drive home here is this: Do not underestimate the power of hope, dreams, goals, or their purpose in healing. They are as essential to the restoration of Mitochondrial populations as any nutrient or exercise. Your Mitochondria will work for you for a lifetime if you treat them as they deserve to be treated—by giving them something to work for, and something to work with. Every moment that you spend in pursuit of your dreams gives your Mitochondria a reason to produce energy. Every time you give your Mitochondria the nutrients, space, and movement they need, they will return the favor with sustained ATP production. That's the promise that Mitochondria offer you. As with any relationship, give, and you shall receive.

The Process of ATP Energy Production Simplified

Mitochondria work from a simple principle—they manufacture Adenosine 5' Triphosphate (ATP) from the air we breathe and the food we eat. So let's take our first excursion into the Cycle of Influencing Energy®, and apply what we have learned to the Anatomy of the Cell and the Mitochondria living within.

ANATOMY OF THE CELL

Each cell of your body is made up of three distinct regions—Cell Wall (Phospholipid Bi-layer), Cell Water (Cytosol), Cell Brain (Nucleus) (See **Figure 4.2** on the next page). The Cell Wall, like any wall, is designed to keep substances out. The Cell Water is designed to promote energy production, protein synthesis, enzyme production, and is designed to detoxify the cell. The Cell Brain tells everything what to do, and when to do it. The region we are interested in is the Cell Water, where all the little cellular organelles live—including populations of Mitochondria. Take note of additional organelles like the Smooth Endoplasmic Reticulum and the Lysosomes. We'll talk more about these in future chapters (they're really, really cool).

ANATOMY OF THE MITOCHONDRIA

Mitochondria have two distinct regions—the Matrix and the Inner Membrane (See **Figure 4.3** on the next page). The Matrix houses the DNA for each Mitochondria, while the Inner Membrane is where ATP is manufactured with the help of specific enzymes. What's interesting about the Inner Membrane of the Mitochondria is that it is composed of a group of chemicals called cytochromes. We will reference cytochromes again when we discuss detoxification, but know for now that cytochromes are made up of porphyrin rings.

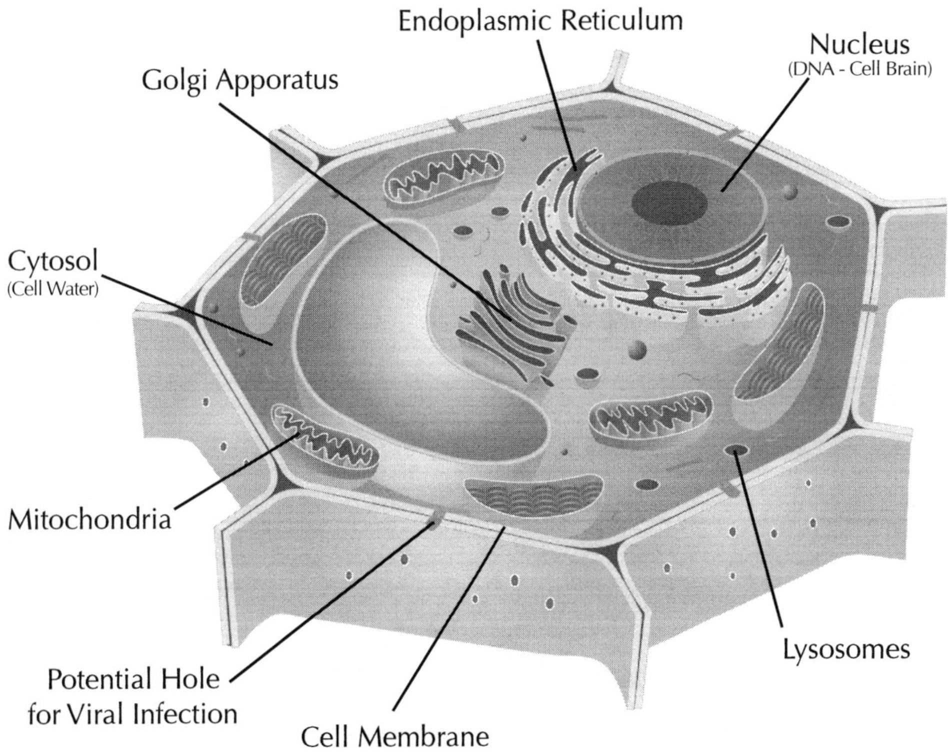

Figure 4.2
Liver Cell. Notice the Mitochondria. Mitochondrial populations will average between 200 and 400 per cell for most cell types.

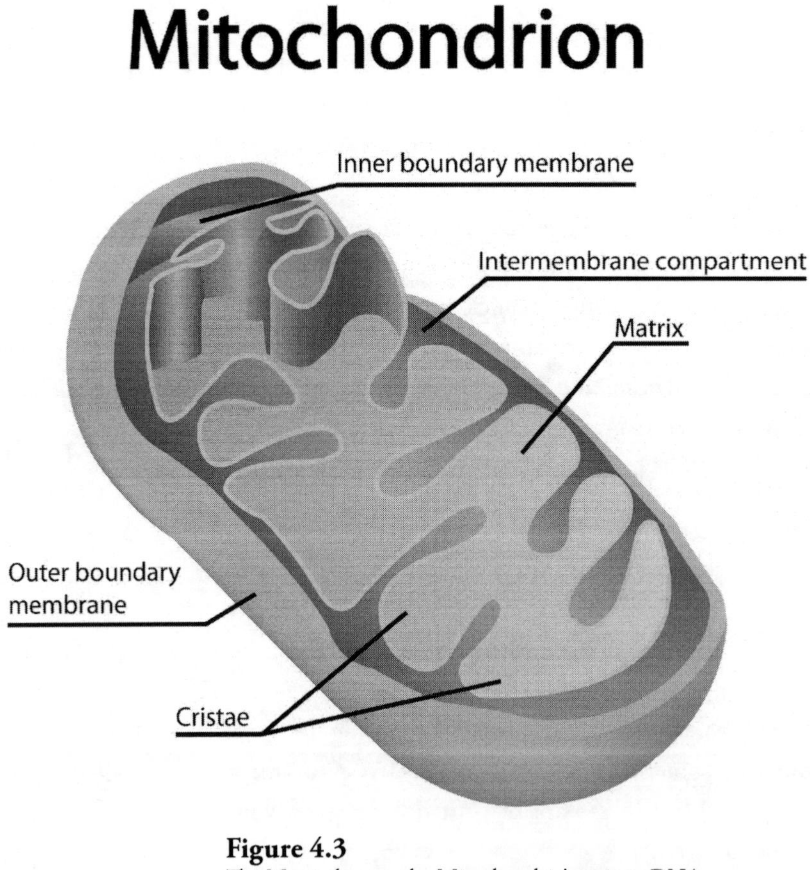

Figure 4.3
The Matrix houses the Mitochondria's unique DNA.

Porphyrin rings can be found abundantly in chlorophyll, so eating something green every day helps your Mitochondria to produce energy and detoxify your body. So understanding the Mitochondria can help us understand the essential relationship between energy production and cellular detoxification.

PHYSIOLOGY OF THE MITOCHONDRIA

The function of the Mitochondria is to produce energy from the air we breathe, and also from the food we eat. When we breathe clean air and consume clean, Organic nutrient-dense foods, we give our Mitochondria the best possible opportunity to cultivate energy. On the flip side, when we breathe in polluted air (including cigarette smoke) and we eat chemically polluted foods, what do you suspect will be the result?

Remember that environmental pollution is a stressor that can creat Acidic Cellular Environments for the Mitochondria. If you'll recall, Mitochondrial Energy Production thrives in an alkaline pH of approximately 7.5. Therefore, environmental pollution—due to its acidic nature—will lower the pH below 7.5, making the Cell Water more acidic. Acidic Cellular Environments make it that much more difficult for Mitochondria to produce energy because they cause damage to the Mitochondria and other organelles living within.

BIOCHEMISTRY OF ENERGY PRODUCTION

The production of ATP can be separated into four unique sequential processes, occurring within the Cell Water and the Mitochondrion (See **Figures 4.4 and 4.5** on the next page).

Glycolysis is a series of nine biotransformations of glucose into various glucose derivatives, ending with Pyruvate. The process of Glycolysis occurs in the Cell Water in preparation for energy precursors like NADH to be supplied to the Electron Transport Chain within the Mitochondrion. Pyruvate is interesting because if your Mitochondrial populations are too low or inefficient, then Pyruvate will convert to lactic acid, which is experienced as a burning sensation during exercise.

Have you ever wondered why some people seem to have great endurance while others fatigue so quickly? Or have you ever wondered what's happening in your body when your endurance changes from day to day? The answer is in the populations and biochemical efficiency of the Mitochondria.

If Mitochondrial populations are low, and/or if Mitochondria do not have all the nutrients they need to produce energy, then their efficiency will suffer. The result is that Pyruvate accumulates in the cytosol and converts over to lactic acid. If this happens quickly during exercise, it is a strong indication of a significant inefficiency in Mitochondrial Energy Production. So how do you know your Mitochondrial populations are growing and becoming more efficient? You have greater endurance in all activities—from exercise to concentration to sexual performance.

But wait—there's more.

Stage	Name	Occurs In
1	**Glycolysis**	Cell Water
2	**PDH Complex**—Pyruvate Dehydrogenase Complex	Mitochondria Matrix
3	**TCA Cycle**—Citric Acid Cycle	Mitochondria Matrix
4	**ETC**—Electron Transport Chain	Mitochondria Inner Membrane

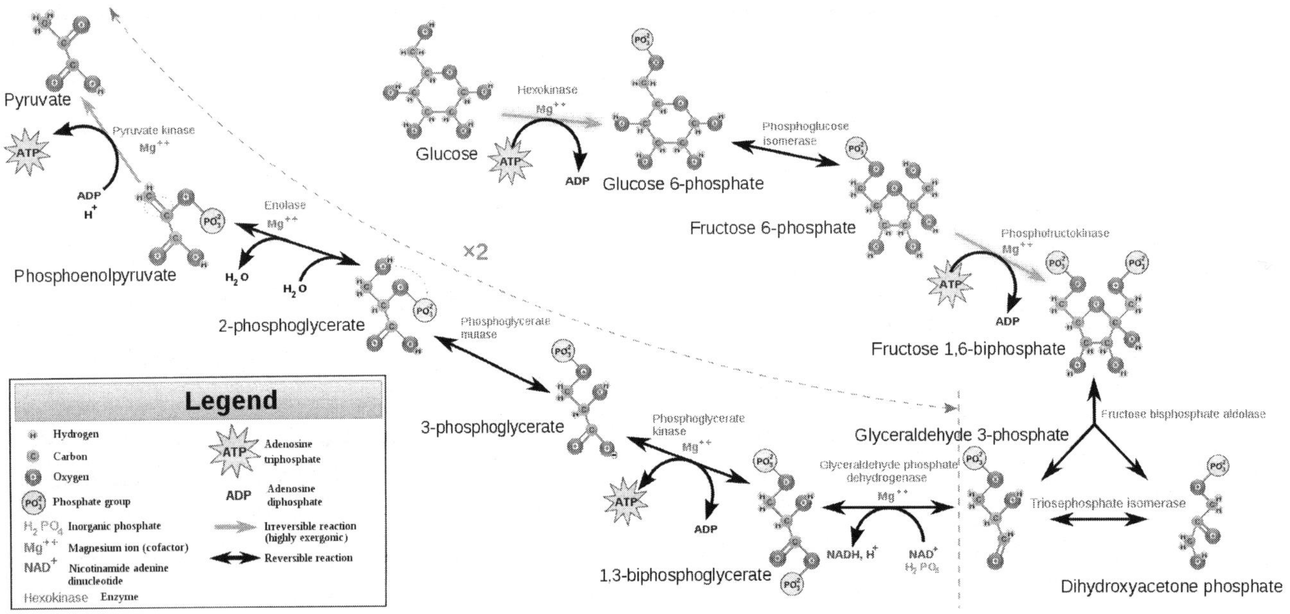

Figure 4.4
Glycolysis. Very easy to get lost in this picture, so don't. The starting point is glucose. The ending point is Pyruvate. And the lesson is that it takes energy to make energy. Simple as that.

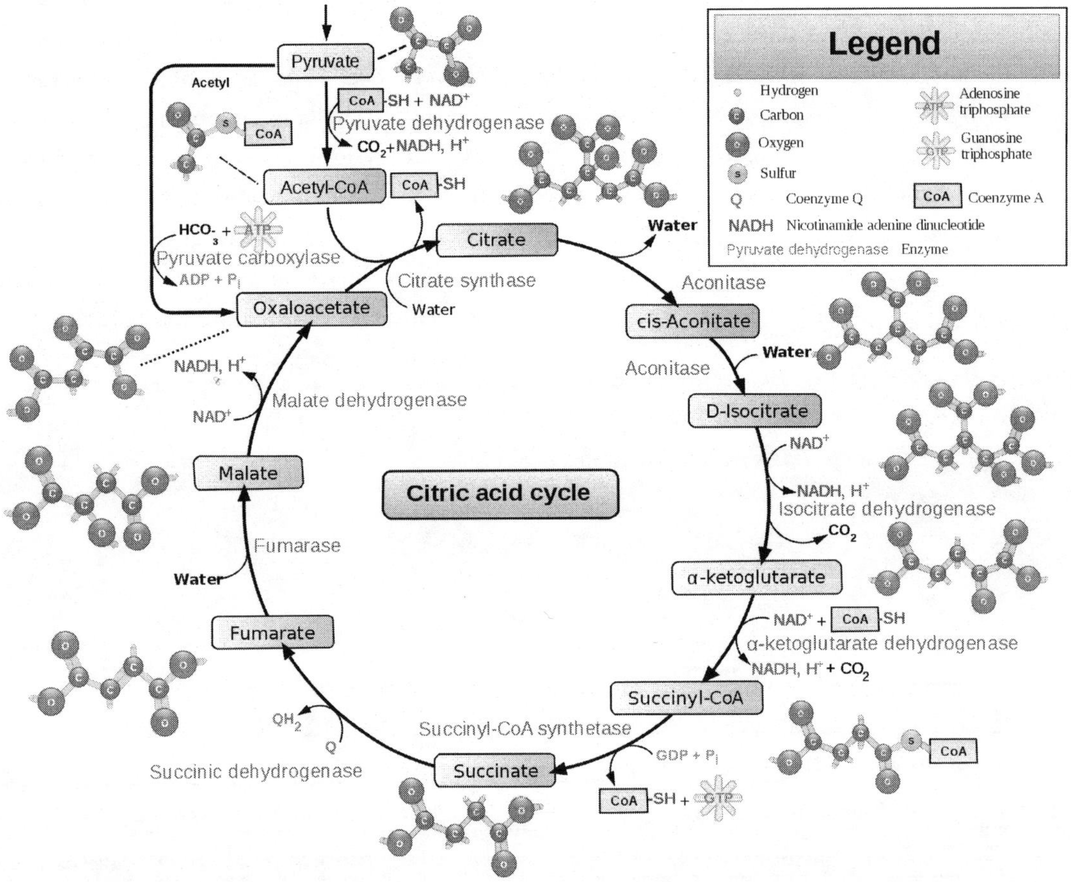

Figure 4.5
TCA Cycle aka Citric Acid Cycle. Very easy to get lost in this picture as well, so go ahead if you'd like to, I have. Or keep it simple. Starting point is Pyruvate from Glycolysis. And the job is to make as much NADH and FADH as possible. The 'H' in NADH and FADH is a hydrogen proton that will help the Mitochondria make ATP.

After Glycolysis, Pyruvate is biotransformed into Acetyl coenzyme A by the three enzymes of the PDH Complex for the next stage of energy production, the TCA Cycle. What's important to know is that both the PDH Complex and the TCA Cycle are similar to Glycolysis in that each of these three stages have a role in biotransforming glucose into the biochemicals essential for energy production, NADH and FADH. NADH and FADH are utilized by the Electron Transport Chain in the final assembly of ATP. So stages 1, 2, and 3 are responsible for generating NADH and FADH. While stage 4 is responsible for utilizing NADH and FADH to assemble ATP. In all—from start to finish—there are as many as thirty-three steps for the energy production of one molecule of ATP from glucose.

It is estimated that one molecule of glucose can generate between thirty and thirty-eight molecules of ATP through the process of Mitochondrial Energy Production. So let's look at some interesting insights. It is estimated that a healthy person—under normal circumstances—can produce between 55 to 60 percent their body weight in ATP every day. That means that a person who weighs 180 pounds will make approximately 108 pounds of ATP every day. Of course if this person is creating an optimal environment for energy production, this number will go up and their demand for it will go down creating a daily surplus. How would it feel if, for example, you were making AND saving $10,000 every day? Conversely, if you are under a significant amount of stress from a variety of sources relative to the 4 Considerations for Healing, then this number will plummet and fatigue will be the end result. So how would you feel if you learned that you were only making $50, while you were wasting more than $100 every day? Cultivation or waste, surplus or deficit—these are the choices before you every day of your life, and for that matter, every moment. Some new age concepts get a bad reputation because they are poorly understood and utilized. Awareness—of which so many people often speak—is one of them. The purpose of awareness does not end with the recognition of a problem. Awareness is an integral aspect of discernment, and therefore, it highlights the necessity for making good decisions in every area of your life.

ADDITIONAL INSIGHTS INTO THE BIOCHEMISTRY OF ENERGY PRODUCTION

Now, I have some additional information that I can't resist sharing with you. Earlier we said that the body has between fifty and seventy-five trillion cells, and that each of these cells have between one and ten thousand Mitochondria. If we average out this range, a good estimate of Mitochondria population per cell is between two hundred and four hundred. We also noted that the typical person—in less than optimal circumstances—can generate approximately 55 to 60 percent of their body weight in ATP every day. For the sake of developing an appreciation of your amazing body, let's apply this information.

I used to wonder how long it would take for one molecule of ATP to be assembled. Thanks to a colleague of mine, I now have way to determine a reasonable answer. My colleague estimates that your body has the ability—in ideal circumstances—to assemble ATP at a rate of 5.50×10^{20} molecules per second. If we say that a person has fifty trillion cells and an average of two hundred Mitochondria per cell, then this gives us an estimated total number of Mitochondria throughout the body that is equivalent to 1.0×10^{16}. If we then say that each of these Mitochondria have to go through thirty-three steps to assemble one molecule of ATP, then this gives us the total number of steps for energy production for each Mitochondria in each cell of your body. The total number of steps at any given moment for energy production throughout the body is around 3.3×10^{17}.

Dividing this number by the rate of ATP production, we get an interesting answer. It takes one Mitochondrion approximately 0.0006 seconds (0.6 milliseconds) to assemble one molecule of ATP.

Topic	Range
Speed of ATP production.	0.6—1.8 milliseconds
Estimated energy produced throughout your body every blink of an eye.	1.83—5.50 x 10^{23} Molecules of ATP
Estimated number of biochemical reactions throughout your body for energy production every blink of an eye.	3.3—9.9 x 10^{20} Biochemical Reactions
ATP produced per second.	5.50 x 10^{20} ATP molecules per second
ATP produced per day.	55—60% of your body weight

Let me put this into perspective for you. Blink your eyelids. Yes, I am asking you to blink your eyelids. ☺ A blink of an eye takes about six hundred milliseconds, about one thousand times slower than it takes for you to make ATP. That's right—blinking an eye is one thousand times slower than energy production. So every time you blink, you are generating at least 5.50 x 10^{23} molecules of ATP. Astounding. *Check out some other calculations above and tell me your body is not beautiful.*

So let me sum the Biochemistry of energy production up using zeros. Every time you blink an eye, your body goes through as many as 990,000,000,000,000,000,000 biochemical reactions in order to produce 550,000,000,000,000,000,000,000 molecules of ATP for energy. That's to say nothing of additional number of incalculable biochemical reactions that your body is initiating every time you blink.

And you want to use this energy for complaining? For lacking faith in the perfection of life? For doubting your own beauty or your worth? Your body is this amazing creation of pure energy, and you want to fuel it with garbage, underuse it, and then get mad at it when it doesn't perform? You've been given everything you need to cultivate the energy you need to realize your dreams, and you want someone to hand life to you? It would seem to me that if you're living in a body, then life has already been handed to you—all you have to do is grab it.

NUTRIENTS FOR ENERGY PRODUCTION

Each stage of energy production requires certain nutrients to act as cofactors for the chain of events to continue. Without any of the nutrients listed below, the process of ATP assembly screeches to a halt.

In addition to the essential nutrients listed below, there are a host of additional nutrients, botanical medicines, and hormones that either make the production of ATP more efficient, more abundant, or help grow Mitochondrial populations per cell. In the table on the next page, the ***bold and italicized*** items have been proven through clinical research to activate the expression of PCG-1α (peroxisome proliferator-activated receptor gamma coactivator 1-alpha). PCG-1α is the key biochemical ingredient responsible for increasing the efficiency, growth, and replication associated with increases in Mitochondrial populations, and as a result, ATP synthesis. A body that has achieved optimal Mitochondrial efficiency and

Nutrients Essential for ATP Assembly

Stage	Name	Nutrients Required
1	Glycolysis	Glucose, Phosphorus, Magnesium, Vitamin B3
2	PDH Complex	Pyruvate, Vitamins B1, B2, B3, B5, Alpha-Lipoic Acid
3	TCA Cycle	Acetyl Coenzyme A, Acetyl L-Carnitine, Vitamins B1, B2, B5,Phosphorus, Magnesium, Alpha-Ketogluterate
4	ETC	Oxygen, NADH and FADH, Vitamin B2, Iron, Sulfur, Copper, Phosphorus, Coenzyme Q 10, D-Ribose

population density per cell will be able to accomplish two very important functions—the maintenance of optimal pH levels for the large variety of cellular function, and the heightened production of cellular enzymes essential for energy production, metabolic function, cellular repair, cellular replication, and cellular detoxification.

ENERGETICS OF MITOCHONDRIA

Now, let's get a little esoteric with all of this for a second. Using the Cycle of Influencing Energy®, we have previously discussed that Anatomy influences Physiology, which influences Biochemistry, which influences Energetics, which influences emotion, and emotion goes full circle to influence Anatomy. The point of using such a thought process is to show how so many things are similar. The Cycle of Influencing Energy® is a way of unifying seemingly divergent concepts—like Western and Eastern medicine—without discounting the validity of either.

Throughout this chapter, we have discussed Mitochondria and ATP. This is an appropriate time to remind you that regardless of whether we say ATP, *Chi*, *Prana*, or the *Vis Medicatrix Naturae*, we are actually describing the exact same thing—we are discussing energy.

It is tempting to say that energy is contained exclusively within each cell, and as such, cannot flow throughout your body. But if that is the case, what are your nerves and blood vessels for then? There is a great saying in Chinese Medicine: *Wherever blood flows, Chi goes.* In Chinese Medicine the two are connected because cells cannot develop ATP without the delivery of nutrients and oxygen from the bloodstream. So before we fully enter into the fascinating world of meridian energy pathways and Energetics at the end of Volume 1 of this text, let's begin our understanding of Energetics with simplicity. While energy does have a physical form in ATP, it also has an auric field—like a shadow of energy—that allows it to move throughout the body. This brings us to **Principle of Advanced Natural Medicine #7:** *Energy will always go first where it is needed most. Your body—in its divine intelligence—has the ability to prioritize between immediately essential and secondarily essential functions.*

EMOTION OF MITOCHONDRIA

It is very, very simple from here. Refer to **Figure 2.2** again. Energy-Draining Reactions cause energy loss, and are a sign of decline in Mitochondrial populations and efficiency. Energy-Cultivating Responses are a result of energy gains, and also signs that Mitochondrial populations are growing and becoming more efficient.

Nutrients and Cofactors Essential for Optimizing Energy Production

Nutrients	Vitamins B6, B12, Folate, Biotin, Selenium, Calcium, Zinc, Potassium, Manganese and Assorted Trace Minerals for the production of Superoxide Dismutase, Chlorophyll, ***Resveratrol, Quercetin, Pyrroloquinoline quinine (PQQ)***, Vitamins A, C, D, E, N-Acetyl Cysteine, Tyrosine, Taurine
Botanicals	***Eleuthrocossus senticosus***, Cordyceps sinensis, Astragalus membranaceus, Camellia sinensis, Glycyrrhiza glabra
Hormones	Insulin, Cortisol, Thyroid Hormone (T_3 and T_4)
Lifestyles	Any physical ***exercise longer than thirty minutes from the point of initial perspiration*** practiced four to six times per week. ***Calorie-Restricted Diets.***

What Stresses Out Your Mitochondria?

In the previous chapter, you learned that your body perceives stress in a much broader way than what we have given if credit for. You also learned that there are four major categories of stress known as the 4 Considerations for Healing—Emotional Charge, Acidic Cellular Environments, Biomechanical Misalignments, and Scar Tissue. Finally, you learned that all stressors lead to the creation of an Acidic Cellular Environment, and that all acid causes damage.

As this pertains to your Mitochondria, understand that stress directly impacts the four stages of energy production—especially the Electron Transport Chain.

Stressor	**Consideration for Healing**	**Effect on Mitochondria**
Energy-Draining Emotions	Emotional Charge	Force Mitochondria to produce energy that is wasted on muscle tension and nerve stimulation.
Poor Posture	Biomechanical Misalignments	Inhibit breathing capacity. As a result, the delivery of oxygen to the Mitochondria essential for energy production.
Old Injuries or Surgeries	Scar Tissue	Constricts blood flow to cells, limiting delivery of nutrients and oxygen essential for Mitochondrial Energy Production.
Antacids (PPIs), Food Preservatives, Pesticides, Herbicides, PCBs, Antibiotics, Barbiturates, Polyaromatic Hydrocarbons (Smoking, CO_2 gas, car exhausts), Cyanide, Plastics, Formaldehyde, **Heavy Metals** (Methylmercury, Mercury, Aluminum, Cadmium, Lead, Arsenic, Thallium)	Acidic Cellular Environments	Breakdown the Electron Transport Chain of the Mitochondria where ATP is assembled. The process is known as decoupling of the cytochrome complexes.
DNA Viral Infections, Trans-Fatty Acids	Acidic Cellular Environments	Breakdown the Electron Transport Chain of the Mitochondria where ATP is assembled.
Alcohol	Acidic Cellular Environments	Depletes body of essential B complex vitamins for ATP production.
THC (Marijuana)	Acidic Cellular Environments	Causes a disruption of the TCA Cycle and Electron Transport Chain, leading to diminished production of ATP.
Fluoride	Acidic Cellular Environments	Covalently binds Magnesium, rendering it unavailable for Glycolysis and the TCA Cycle.
Nutrient Deficiencies, Hypothyroidism, Adrenal Fatigue	Acidic Cellular Environments	Prevent various stages of the energy-production process from working efficiently, leading to fatigue.

So with the chart on the previous page, let's take a look at some of the specific stressors that impact your Mitochondria, and what effect they have on them.

Of particular interest to me are antacids, because I want to create an argument against their long-term use. Most new classes of antacids are categorized as Proton Pump Inhibitors (PPIs). PPIs work by essentially turning off the proton pumps in the stomach that allow for the production of a very essential enzyme called hydrochloric acid. As PPIs pertain to your Mitochondria, it is important to note that the Electron Transport Chain uses proton pumps in the final assembly of ATP along the Inner Membrane. Protons are labeled H+ (See **Figure 4.6** on the next page). Therefore, I would like you to be aware that PPIs may be doing more than just turning off stomach acid. They also may be decoupling the cytochromes of the Electron Transport Chain, and as a result, creating a tremendous obstacle to energy production.

PPIs also have the potential of disrupting Lysosomal activity within immune cells. We will discuss this in more detail when we cover the Immune System in Volume 2.

Preliminary Notes on Cortisol and Thyroid Hormones

At this point you may be thinking to yourself: *Why have I never heard of cortisol before? I've heard about the thyroid, but not much about cortisol.* So what are the implications for your Mitochondria?

Hormones are a critical means of communication between various systems in the body. In essence, they are chemical messengers that stimulate or stop specific cellular functions. In doing so, they allow the target cells to participate in maintaining homeostasis within the body. Looking more closely within the cell, hormones help to stimulate or stop specific cellular functions by helping to regulate enzyme production. Enzymes are protein-based structures that accelerate biochemical conversions, and as you learned earlier, time is of the essence in this process. Imagine trying to assemble a molecule of ATP through a thirty-three-step process every 0.6 of a millisecond without the help of enzymes.

All cell life is, energy and enzyme dependent, meaning that energy supports the production of enzymes, while enzymes allow for the production of energy—in addition to a number of other functions.

Thyroid hormone and cortisol are both essential components of the Mitochondrial energy-production process. If glucose is the fuel for energy production, then thyroid hormone and cortisol create the fire that helps the Mitochondria burn the fuel and convert it into ATP. If the presence of either hormone is deficient, then the Mitochondria will adapt by utilizing more of the available hormone. So, for example, if your body is deficient in thyroid hormone, then it can compensate by using more cortisol, and vice versa. However, this compensation is not without a price. A deficiency of thyroid hormone can lead to a temporary overproduction of cortisol. Much like burning the candle at both ends, any overproduction can lead to glandular fatigue. Without fire to burn the fuel, energy production becomes woefully inefficient, and Mitochondrial populations dwindle. And how is this all experienced?

It's as if your get up and go, got up and went. Some of the signs of low cortisol levels include fatigue, diminished desire without cause, difficulty waking up in the morning, falling asleep during the day, weight gain, sexual dysfunction, lack of interest in activities, and other symptoms. The signs for low thyroid hormone are very similar. Some of the symptoms include fatigue, weight gain, brittle hair and nails, feeling cold, and Skin that is dry and has lost its vitality. These are just a few of the early warning signs that your body may not have what it needs to produce energy.

There are two important ideas to understand at this point. First, fatigue hampers the body's ability to detoxify, and the end result is Bio-accumulation. Secondly—and I can't emphasize this enough—your body can recover as long as enough viable glandular tissue is available.

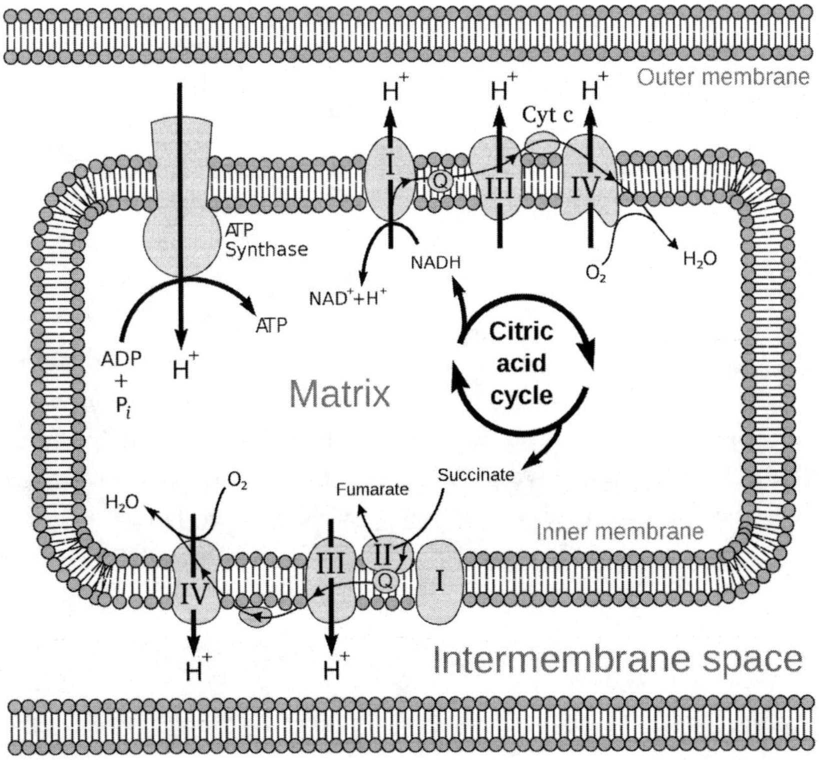

Figure 4.6 A
Electron Transport Chain. This picture demonstrates where the Citric Acid Cycle occurs in the Matrix of the Mitochondria and where the Electron Transport Chain occurs along the Inner Membrane of the Mitochondria. Notice the little H+'s. These are hydrogen protons. Keep it simple.

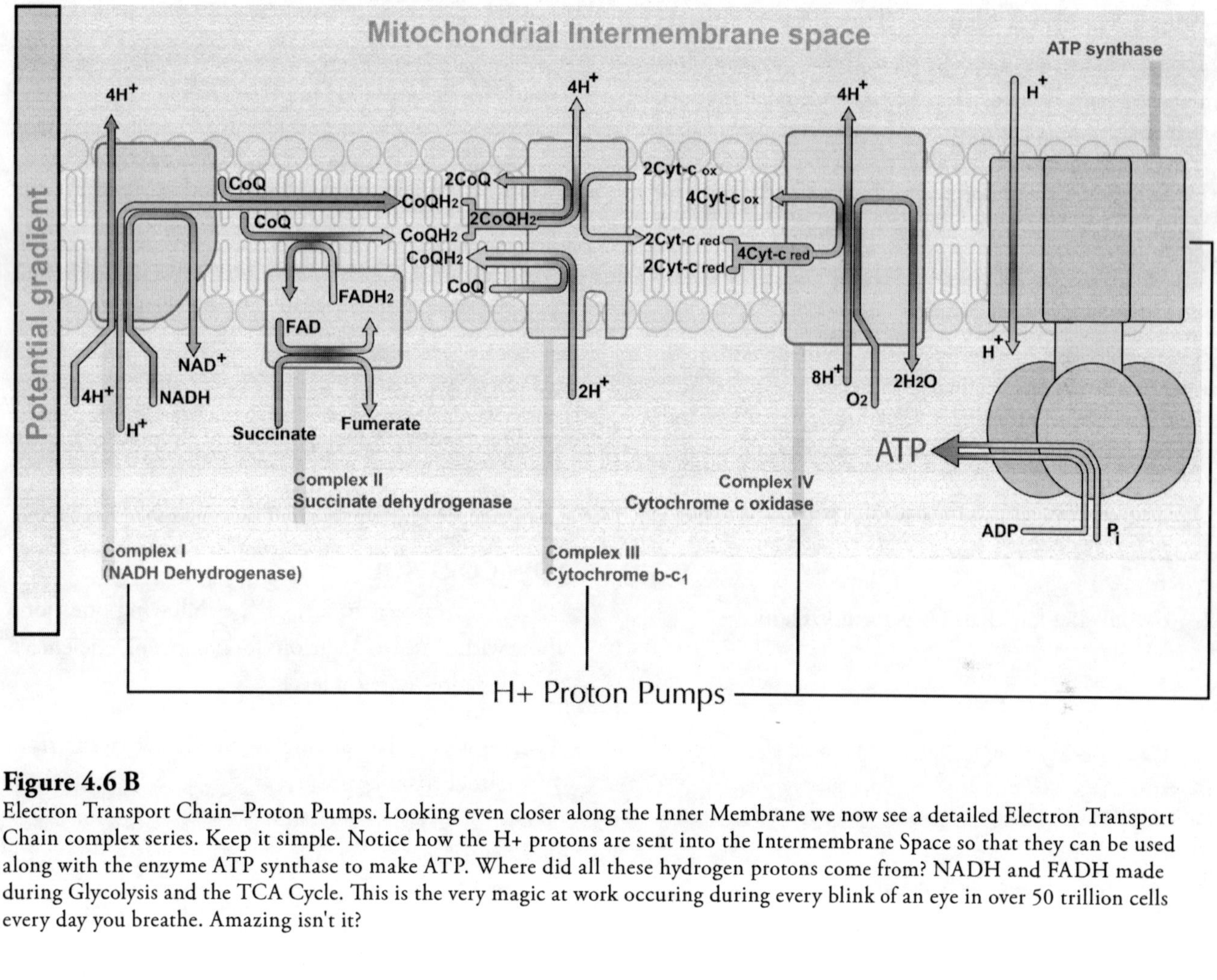

Figure 4.6 B

Electron Transport Chain–Proton Pumps. Looking even closer along the Inner Membrane we now see a detailed Electron Transport Chain complex series. Keep it simple. Notice how the H+ protons are sent into the Intermembrane Space so that they can be used along with the enzyme ATP synthase to make ATP. Where did all these hydrogen protons come from? NADH and FADH made during Glycolysis and the TCA Cycle. This is the very magic at work occuring during every blink of an eye in over 50 trillion cells every day you breathe. Amazing isn't it?

Listening to Your Amazing Body

When assessing fatigue, it is possible to focus on the likely source of the disruption in energy production, and to assume that nutrient deficiencies are always a factor in the problem. So when you are fatigued, it is always a good idea to supplement your diet with high-quality nutrients at the correct Therapeutic Range (a concept we will discuss in the next chapter). For now, let's investigate the most common suspects—Nutrient Deficiencies, Anemia Blood Deficiencies, Low Cortisol, Low Thyroid Hormone, Sedentary Lifestyles, Environmental Pollution, Viral Infection, and Emotional Charge. Below are a series of questions designed to help you focus on the likely sources of disruption in the energy-production process within your body.

NUTRIENT DEFICIENCIES

A 'Yes' answer to any of the following questions suggests a nutrient deficiency.

1. Are you frequently fatigued, exhausted, or unenthusiastic?

   Yes No

2. Is your diet less than 80 percent Organic?

   Yes No

3. Is your body slow to heal?

   Yes No

4. Is your urine regularly clear?

   Yes No

5. Do you frequently get sick?

   Yes No

6. Have you been recently diagnosed with any chronic illness?

   Yes No

7. Do you frequently feel stressed out?

   Yes No

8. Do you take antacids (PPIs)?

   Yes No

9. Do you have more than two glasses of alcohol per month?

   Yes No

ANEMIA BLOOD DEFICIENCIES

A 'Yes' answer to any of the following questions, along with a 'Yes' to questions for Nutrient Deficiencies, suggests anemia blood deficiencies.

1. Has recent lab testing revealed an iron deficiency or a vitamin B12/Folate deficiency anemia?

   Yes No

2. Has your Skin lost color, and is it looking dull?

   Yes No

LOW CORTISOL

A 'Yes' answer to any of the following questions, along with a 'Yes' to questions for Nutrient Deficiencies, suggests a low cortisol level.

1. Has recent lab testing revealed low twenty-four hour cortisol levels?

   Yes No

2. Are your total cholesterol levels below 170?

   Yes No

3. Do you sleep through your alarm?

   Yes No

4. Does it take you more than fifteen minutes to wake up and get going?

   Yes No

5. Do you drink several cups of coffee to help you get through your day?

   Yes No

6. Are your joints inflamed or stiff?

   Yes No

7. Do you get less than six hours of sleep each night?

   Yes No

8. Have you gained more than ten pounds even though you exercise?

   Yes No

9. Do you often find yourself on the verge of falling asleep while driving or while at work?

   Yes No

LOW THYROID HORMONE

A 'Yes' answer to any of the following questions, along with a 'Yes' to questions for Nutrient Deficiencies, suggests low thyroid hormone levels.

1. Has recent lab testing revealed imbalances in TSH, Free T_3, Total T_3, Free T_4, Total $T_{4,}$ Thyroid antibodies, or low iodine?

   Yes No

2. Are you frequently cold?

   Yes No

3. Are your hair or nails damaged or brittle?

   Yes No

4. Have you gained more than ten pounds even though you exercise?

   Yes No

5. Is your Skin very dry?

   Yes No

6. Are your reflexes slow or delayed?

   Yes No

7. Do you frequently eat cruciferous vegetables raw (Broccoli, Kale, Bok Choy, Cabbage, Collard Greens, Mustard Greens, Radishes, Turnips, Cauliflower, Arugula, Watercress, Brussel Sprouts)?

   Yes No

SEDENTARY LIFESTYLE

A 'Yes' answer to any of the following questions, along with a 'Yes' to questions for Nutrient Deficiencies, suggests a sedentary lifestyle.

1. Is your resting pulse (Heart Rate) above seventy beats per minute?

   Yes No

2. Have you been diagnosed with Restless Leg Syndrome?

   Yes No

3. Are you easily 'winded' when you begin exercising?

   Yes No

4. Does your body feel soft, droopy, or unattractive?

   Yes No

5. Do you exercise without sweating?

   Yes No

6. Do you exercise less than four times per week for at least thirty minutes after you begin to perspire?

   Yes No

7. Does it take you longer than nine minutes to run a mile?

   Yes No

ENVIRONMENTAL POLLUTION

A 'Yes' answer to any of the following questions, along with a 'Yes' to questions for Nutrient Deficiencies, suggests exposure to environmental pollution. This is a preliminary list we will expand on later when we discuss detoxification.

1. Do you have silver amalgam fillings?

   Yes No

2. Do you eat farm-raised fish?

   Yes No

3. Do you work with chemicals of any kind?

   Yes No

4. Do you keep chemical cleaners or air-fresheners in your home?

   Yes No

5. Does breathing fumes make you feel light-headed?

   Yes No

6. Do you smoke or take recreational drugs?

   Yes No

7. Do you use Fluoride toothpaste or drink tap water?

   Yes No

8. Do you eat non-Organic produce?

   Yes No

9. Do you use weed-killer chemicals?

   Yes No

DNA VIRAL INFECTIONS

A 'Yes' answer to any of the following questions, along with a 'Yes' to questions for Nutrient Deficiencies, suggests DNA viral infections that are not being effectively cleared.

1. Do your muscles frequently ache?

   Yes No

2. Do you find yourself typically running a slight temperature?

   Yes No

3. Are your lymph nodes frequently swollen?

   Yes No

4. Have you been diagnosed with Chronic Fatigue Syndrome?

   Yes No

5. Does your nose run with a clear discharge?

   Yes No

6. Do you have a history of Mono, Herpes, or other viral infection?

   Yes No

EMOTIONAL CHARGE

A 'Yes' answer to the following question, along with a 'Yes' to questions for Nutrient Deficiencies, suggests Emotional Charge.

1. Do you frequently succumb to Energy-Draining Reactions?

   Yes No

WHAT YOU CAN DO TO CULTIVATE ENERGY TODAY

Here are some final thoughts on how to apply the information you have learned so that you can increase your Mitochondrial populations, and also make them more efficient. We've covered stressors that work against the body's ability to produce energy. So removing them—or at least minimizing them—is an excellent start. We've also covered essential nutrients for optimizing energy production. So making sure these are a part of your regular lifestyle is absolutely essential to all Healing Processes. Below is a list of the main factors that are essential for maintaining healthy and happy Mitochondrial populations.

	Good Decisions for Energy Production that Build Momentum
1	**FIND WHAT'S GOOD**—What if you trained yourself to spend more time thinking about What's Good in your life than about what's stressing you out? Every time you think of something stressful, immediately find at least two things that are good. Make the discovery of What's Good an everyday pursuit.
2	**NUTRIENT DELIVERY**—Utilize ***Genesis Therapeutic Range®*** Supplements. **FORMULA 1—ATP ESSENTIALS** AND **FORMULA 2—MITOCHONDRIAL PEAK PERFORMANCE** I have formulated both of these products to deliver the highest-quality nutrients essential for energy production, at the perfect dose for your body's needs. They are designed to make your life easier and to help your body.
3	**EAT SOMETHING ORGANIC AND GREEN EVERY DAY**—Eating Organic food ensures that there are no pesticide residues, and that your food is as nutrient dense as possible. Green ensures that you are eating all the building blocks for porphyrin rings, which are essential to energy production and healthy detoxification. Green also ensures that you are helping your body achieve the alkaline pH essential for optimal energy production.
4	**MOVE YOUR BODY**—Exercising three to five times per week for a minimum of thirty minutes *after* you begin to perspire is a key component of building healthy and happy Mitochondria.
5	**SLEEP**—For reasons we will discuss later (pertaining to cellular replication and restoration), give your body at least eight total hours of sleep each day. Or if this is not possible, choose at least one day per week to sleep until your body is ready to wake up—even if that means sleeping more than ten hours.
6	**HOUSE CLEANING**—Most chemicals have a damaging impact on energy production. Change your household cleaners from chemical-based to natural soaps like Dr. Bronner's. Use every opportunity you have to lower the toxic assault of chemicals on your Mitochondria. Getting rid of pesticides, chemical household cleaners, and amalgam fillings take an enormous burden off your Mitochondria.
7	**GET THE METAL OUT OF YOUR MOUTH**—If you are interested in longevity and great health, then this is an absolute essential part of caring for your long-term health. Get all the silver amalgam fillings in your mouth replaced with composites immediately so that you can remove your daily exposure to mercury. Remember that mercury breaks down the Electron Transport Chain in your Mitochondria.

RESOLUTION #5

In resolution #4, we suggested that you avoid two stressors. Now we want you to select two methods of improving your Mitochondrial Energy Production, and follow the revised Alkalizing Healing Plan for one week. Sometimes the best way to remove stress is to simply focus on things that make you feel good. In other words, don't focus on stress or give it any energy.

Good decisions for energy production that I will use to my advantage this week:

1. ______________________________

2. ______________________________

HEALING JOURNAL RECORDING

Record in your Healing Journal your moods, thoughts, and positive experiences throughout the week, paying particular attention to your focus. Have you spent more time thinking about What's Good?

Good Luck!

ALKALIZING HEALING PLAN

	Therapy	Instructions
Primary Therapy	Organic Clinical Nutrition	Eat something Organic, green and chlorophyll-rich every day; eat 80 percent or more Organic.
Complementary Therapy	Breathing Practice	Upon waking and before starting your morning routine, breathe silently for fifteen to thirty minutes.
Complementary Therapy	Yoga	Activate your feet frequently throughout the day while standing, walking, or sitting.
Complementary Therapy	Exercise	Exercise using whatever method or variety of methods you choose. The goal is a minimum of thirty minutes from the time you begin to perspire, three to five times a week.
Essential Therapy	Sleep	Give yourself either eight hours of sleep every night, or choose one day to sleep for as long as your body needs to sleep.
Essential Therapy	Positive Internal Dialogue	Finding Something Good. Before you go to sleep, reflect on four things that happened during your day that made you feel good. During your day when you find yourself thinking about something stressful, change. Find something good.

CHAPTER 5: THE ART OF EATING HEALTHY

Have You Ever Wondered What Nutrition Really Is?

Interesting Insights to look for in this chapter:

- Pesticides role of destruction upon your Heart, Lungs, and Nervous System.
- A sick body leads to an empty bank account.
- Every 4 grams of refined sugar = 1 teaspoon… that's all your body needs.
- Pus cells and the cow.

Principle of Advanced Natural Medicine #8:

Let Organic food be thy medicine, and thy medicine be Organic food. Organic food tastes better because it is better.

—Hippocrates (Updated with a modern feel)

But I Eat Healthy, Doc

Wow! How many times have I heard that one? If I had a nickel for every time I've heard that, I'd have a whole bunch of nickels.

The first thing that we need to do when discussing nutrition is surrender our pride, the vanity, the standoffishness, and everything that you've heard from a friend of a friend of an uncle's mother's second cousin's next-door neighbor. Remember what we talked about in the first chapter—our society is one of the most undereducated and miseducated when it comes to the body, health, and how to get healthy. It sometimes seems as though there is too much information out there about how to get healthy—and sometimes the information contradicts itself. A very fundamental principle of life that we will apply is the **Principle of Advanced Natural Medicine #9**: *More is not better—better is better.* More information is not necessarily better. More nutrients are not necessarily better. And more Fast-food, pharmaceuticals, refined sugar, and sitting on your rear end are not better—for your emotional state or your body. So let's take a look at what is better.

If we are going to effectively and fully utilize the principles of Advanced Natural Medicine, then no healing plan is complete without a strict attention to what goes into the body. Removing all ambiguity about what Eating Healthy means is essential to making good decisions that will build momentum in your energy production, and ultimately, in your life. Does this make sense? Yes? Then let's move forward.

Many people ask the wrong questions, and in the wrong order when selecting a meal. The internal dialogue probably goes something like this: What do I feel like eating What tastes good? What will take me the least amount of time and effort to pick-up? It's very difficult to Eat? Healthy when you aren't preparing food in your own kitchen. And it's virtually impossible to Eat Healthy when you shop at stores that sell less than 25 percent Organic.

A better question and thought process in selecting food choices is: What's going to make me and my body feel great? There's no second question involved because when you're Eating Healthy, Organic foods already, they taste ridiculously amazing! Now all you have to do is find places to shop that can offer you a good selection of Organic produce and products.

Below is a checklist I developed years ago to help my nutrition students understand that Eating Healthy means much more than choosing chicken over beef on the fast-food menu, or selecting diet soda over regular soda. At first glance, this may seem daunting, but I will help you simplify the thought process behind each aspect of Eating Healthy so that you can immediately put it to tasty good use. Let's have some learning fun.

Eating Healthy Guidelines Checklist		
1	Does your meal proved all the nutrients essential for **Mitochondrial Energy Production**?	✓
2	Is your meal made of **Organic-Sourced Foods for Optimal Nutrient Density**?	✓
3	Is your meal free of known **Delayed Food Allergens**?	✓
4	Is your meal at least **60 percent Alkalizing**?	✓
5	Does your meal have at least **one Green Food**?	✓
6	Is your meal filled with **Oxygen Radical Absorbance Capacity (ORAC) Antioxidants**?	✓
7	Does your meal have less than 8 grams of **Refined Sugar**?	✓
8	Does your meal include something **Naturally Sweet**?	✓
9	Are there 8 to 12 grams of **Total Fiber** in your meal?	✓
10	Does your meal include a **Raw Fruit or Vegetable**?	✓
11	Is your meal prepared using **Healthy Preparation Methods**?	✓
12	Does your meal include **Environmentally Safe Meats and Fish**?	✓
13	Is your meal prepared using **Environmentally Safe Cookware**?	✓
14	Are **Family and Friends** involved in the preparation and cleanup of the meal?	✓
15	Is the **Beverage** you are having with your meal alkalizing and 8 ounces or less?	✓
16	Can you burn off the **Total Calories** in the same day?	✓

STOP! Who in the heck is going to do all of this before eating one meal? It seems sooooooo restrictive. You might be saying to yourself: *I can't do this.*

Well, allow me to retort. Negative internal dialogue can derail positive changes before they even have a chance to take root. Let me ask you a few questions.

Do you want to get the most out of your body, your unique potential, and your life? Yes? Very Good.

Do you want your family members to have every advantage they need in order to realize their dreams? Yes? Great.

Do you want your children to have great attitudes and perform brilliantly in school? Of Course! Fantastic.

Then it sounds like you are going to be exploring these concepts of Eating Healthy with me. Let me make two comments before I begin telling you why these factors are essential for your body.

First of all, these guidelines are not meant to be strict or restrictive. They are meant to be working guidelines for the person who is in charge of a family's day-in-and-day-out eating habits. The guidelines are meant to help educate and establish healthy staples in the diet. And as you read further, you will see that they are designed for family, participation in meal preparation to help foster healthy communication within the family AND to give mom (or dad) a well-deserved break from doing it all.

Second, we all know that regardless of what anyone tells you to do, you are probably going to do what you want to do—and deservedly so. I'm not here to pretend to be holier than thou—I'm here to share ideas that can make your life happier. It may involve a little work to initiate these changes at first. And there may be a little resistance from the family. So what? If the family is happier, healthier, and more together, isn't a little change in the kitchen worth it? In my years of developing and practicing the Eating Healthy thought process I have learned that there are days when I stray from it. And when I do, I find that I pay the price for it. But it's so wonderful to always have something to come back to, when my body, moods, and my life begin to diverge from the wonderful I normally feel. Once you try this for a week or two—if you're like most of my students—you'll really enjoy Eating Healthy— and your family just might surprise you, too.

The Skinny on Eating Healthy

Each of the following aspects of Eating Healthy plays a huge role in energy production, immune function, digestion, and cardiovascular health. Of particular importance are the first sixteen aspects. Just kidding. I couldn't resist. We have a lot of work to do, so let's get started.

MITOCHONDRIAL ENERGY PRODUCTION

As this was the teaching topic for chapter 4, let's review several of keys aspects for growing Mitochondrial populations, and optimizing their production of energy:

- Mitochondria thrive in a stress-free environment (*recall the 4 Considerations for Healing to review how your body perceives stress*).
- Mitochondria thrive in an Alkaline Cellular Environment at or near 7.5 on the pH scale.
- Mitochondria thrive in a body that enjoys frequent cardiovascular activity.
- Mitochondria thrive with a balance of thyroid hormone and cortisol.
- Mitochondria require nutrients that allow them to reach their peak performance, and to produce ATP.

The production of energy at the Mitochondrial level is the first and most important consideration for Eating Healthy and achieving optimal health. If you have a deficiency of any of the following nutrients in your meal, or if the nutrients are insufficient for your body's Therapeutic Range of needs, then you will you will be more likely to overconsume expensive, empty calories. On the next page are two tables of nutrients from chapter 4.

Nutrients Essential for ATP Assembly

Stage	Name	Nutrients Required
1	Glycolysis	Glucose, Phosphorus, Magnesium, Vitamin B3
2	PDH Complex	Pyruvate, Vitamins B1, B2, B3, B5, Alpha-Lipoic Acid
3	TCA Cycle	Acetyl Coenzyme A, Acetyl L-Carnitine, Vitamins B1, B2, B5,Phosphorus, Magnesium, Alpha-Ketogluterate
4	ETC	Oxygen, NADH and FADH, Vitamin B2, Iron, Sulfur, Copper, Phosphorus, Coenzyme Q 10, D-Ribose

Nutrients and Cofactors Essential for Optimizing Energy Production

Nutrients	Vitamins B6, B12, Folate, Biotin, Selenium, Calcium, Zinc, Potassium, Manganese and Assorted Trace Minerals for the production of Superoxide Dismutase, Chlorophyll, ***Resveratrol, Quercetin, Pyrroloquinoline quinine (PQQ)***, Vitamins A, C, D, E, N-Acetyl Cysteine, Tyrosine, Taurine
Botanicals	***Eleuthrocossus senticosus***, Cordyceps sinensis, Astragalus membranaceus, Camellia sinensis, Glycyrrhiza glabra
Hormones	Insulin, Cortisol, Thyroid Hormone (T_3 and T_4)
Lifestyles	Any physical ***exercise longer than thirty minutes from the point of initial perspiration*** practiced four to six times per week. ***Calorie-Restricted Diets.***

The following is a final thought on the relationship between Mitochondria and herbs. **Principle of Advanced Natural Medicine #10**: *Botanical Medicines reach their peak effectiveness when Mitochondria have everything they require to produce energy.*

ORGANIC-SOURCED FOODS FOR OPTIMAL NUTRIENT DENSITY

A chilling reality of the chemical revolution since World War II is that as of 2010 an estimated five billion pounds of pesticide are currently being produced every year to satisfy demand worldwide. As insects become more resistant to pesticides, harsher pesticides are developed and an unwinnable battle continues that ultimately pollutes our food supply. Of the five billion (that's 5,000,000,000,000) pounds of pesticide produced annually, the United States is responsible for using more than one billion pounds annually. This is equivalent to nearly four pounds of pesticide for every man, woman, and child in the United States. As of 2010, the world is comprised of 195 independent nations, and the United States uses and consumes roughly 20 percent of all the pesticide produced in the world each year. How can this *not* result in imbalance and a decline in the health of our population?

It is interesting to me that once upon a time, this great nation was considered a world leader where environmental policies were concerned, and that it prospered from the lowest percentage of Gross Domestic Product spent on healthcare. The last great era of tangible prosperity our country enjoyed was from 1901 to 1909 while Theodore Roosevelt was president. It is no coincidence that following World War II, several factors led to our current state of ill health—economically and as a society. Chief among these factors is the increasing use of pesticides in our food supply. However, our undereducation, miseducation, and lack of appreciation for our bodies and our health also have played a significant role in the decline of our overall health. When you consider our overconsumption of refined sugars, our overreliance on antibiotics and antacids, our reduction in sleep hours, our lack of exercise, our increased stress levels, and the diseases and outcomes that result from these decisions, it's not difficult to understand why we are experiencing a decline in our physical health and in our economy. As of 2010, the outcome of each of these cofactors is a nation of illness where we spend a higher percentage of Gross Domestic Product (GDP) than *any other nation on the planet. Meaning we rank last in the world in terms of healthcare.*

Experts at the World Health Organization estimate that a healthy nation spends between 3 and 4 percent of its GDP on healthcare, which includes government spending, private party/company spending, and out-of-pocket spending. What this means is that each person should spend, on average, 3 and 4 percent or less than what they earn in annual gross income on healthcare if they plan to enjoy financial prosperity in their lives.

Guess what percentage of GDP the United States spends on healthcare? Between 2000 and 2010, the United States spent between 14 and 16 percent of its GDP on healthcare. This confirms several realities:

- We are a sick nation.
- We have a healthcare system that is broken.
- We have a healthcare system that is woefully inefficient.
- It is our collective fault.

For historical reference, the United States spent under less than 1 percent of its GDP on healthcare (see **Figure 5.1**). At that time, we were ranked #1 in the world in healthcare and this was one of the main reasons why our great nation was so attractive to people hoping to immigrate from other countries. Now, it would seem that most people are attracted to our country because of the free ride that our government services seem to provide, rather than on the freedoms that initially attracted so many immigrants in the early history of the nation. You and I have the ability to change this by more carefully considering what we allow in our kitchens. What a novel concept!

Now, take another look at the percent of GDP Spent on Healthcare chart. Notice how our country was relatively stable from 1901 until about 1966. After that period, there was a steady rise in healthcare spending. So what happened in 1966? What changed? By 1966, we saw the rise of the fast-food industry, and along with it, were proportional rises in the consumption of calories, refined sugar, sodium, and saturated animal fat. We also saw the entire food industry change to meet public demand. This change included the shift to monoculture crops (i.e. russet potatoes for french fry demand), as well as the increases in pesticides, herbicides, confined animal feeding operations, the use of antibiotics, growth hormones in meats, and the accompanying increases in overweight, obese, and morbidly obese Americans.

As noted in Eric Schlosser's book, *Fast-food Nation*, "In 1970, Americans spent about $6 billion on Fast-food; in 2000, they spent more than $110 billion. Americans now spend more money on Fast-food than on higher education, personal computers, computer software, or new cars. They spend more on Fast-food than on movies, books, magazines, newspapers, videos, and recorded music—combined."

This is what we call a major problem. Thankfully, we can do something about the problem.

The point I am hoping to drive home is this: A sick body leads to individual financial disaster, and a nation of sick bodies also leads our great nation to the brink of disaster. As unthinkable as it is, our healthcare system (and desire to wage never-ending wars that return no resources to our country) is likely to bankrupt our nation and set our dollar up for a free fall. *So is the key to reform the healthcare system, or reform the body so that there is less of a need to access the healthcare system?* I'm no politician or economist, but I do know that a person in great health does not need to visit the doctor as often, and the money they save can be spent on American-made products (if they

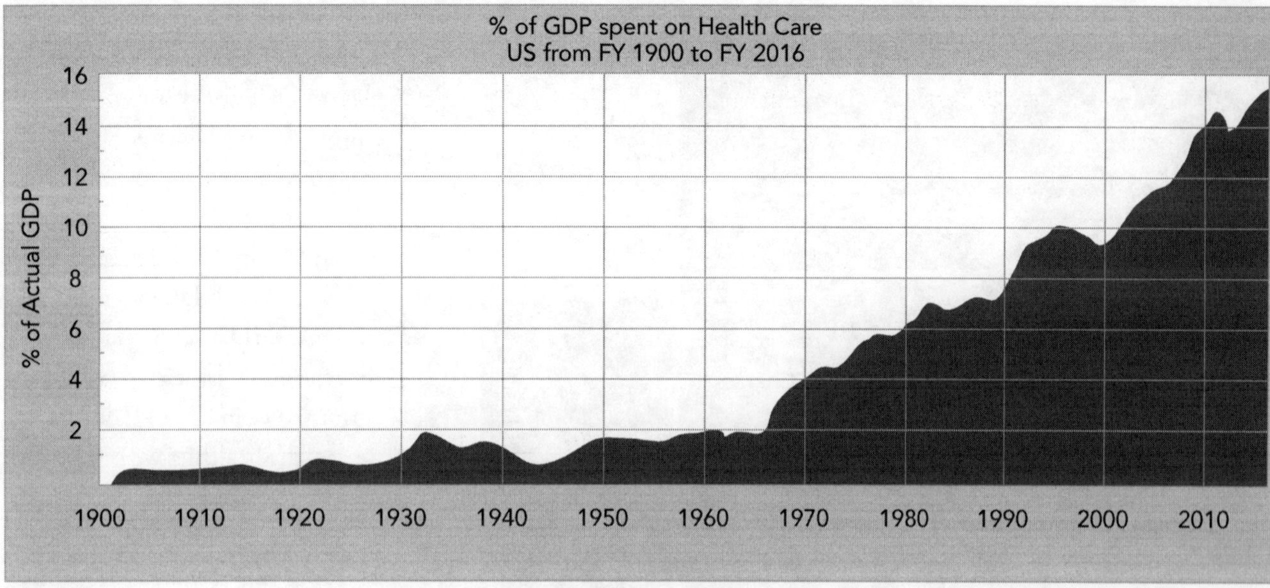

Figure 5.1
Notice the spike around 1966 as the Fast-food Industry grows to meet demand. The most important question is what's different between 1910 and 2010? Calorie Consumption has increased. Trans Fatty Acids and Saturated Animal Fats have increased. Environmental Pollution has increased. Antibiotic Consumption has increased. Overall stress to the body has increased. While sleep and a sense of security have decidedly decreased.

exist anymore). Eating Healthy provides a solution to issues that have an impact on our country's future, while also allowing you to buy local and American. Eating Healthy builds our economy on a multitude of levels, and it tastes good too. But let's get back to why pesticides are bad for your body.

The top four leading causes of death in the United States as of 2007 are: Heart Disease (616,067), Cancer (562,875), Stroke (135,952), Chronic Lower Respiratory Disease (127,924). Notice the huge gaps between heart disease, cancer, and stroke. Really we have two leading causes of death. What you need to know is that pesticides and all environmental pollutants are directly linked to each of these leading causes of death. Let's learn how.

Pesticides are classified into several categories of environmental pollutants. These include organophosphates, organochlorines, and acetylcholine esterase inhibitors. Most people do not know how pesticides kill insects. The majority of pesticides work by significantly disrupting the Nervous System, and as a result, heart rhythm and respiration. Acetylcholine Esterase Inhibitors—which will be our focus because they make up the majority of pesticides—literally inhibit the enzyme known as acetylcholine esterase, causing the insect to suffocate while having a heart attack.

So let's back up for a second and talk about the importance of acetylcholine esterase in the insect's Nervous System. An insect's Nervous System works using acetylcholine as the predominant neurotransmitter, meaning that acetylcholine is how one nerve communicates to another. This is best witnessed in the insect's brain, using acetylcholine to tell its lungs to breath and its heart to beat. As with any communication through the Nervous System, a stop signal must come through to tell the lungs to relax and exhale, and the heart to relax and fill with blood before it pumps again. Acetylcholine esterase is an enzyme that acts like an eraser, clearing the space between neighboring neurons of any acetylcholine that has accumulated in the space (See **Figure 5.2**).

So in essence, acetylcholine is the green light, and acetylcholine esterase is the red light. In order for the insect's body to work properly—in order for it to be able to breathe and for its heart to beat—it needs the green light and then the red light so that the green

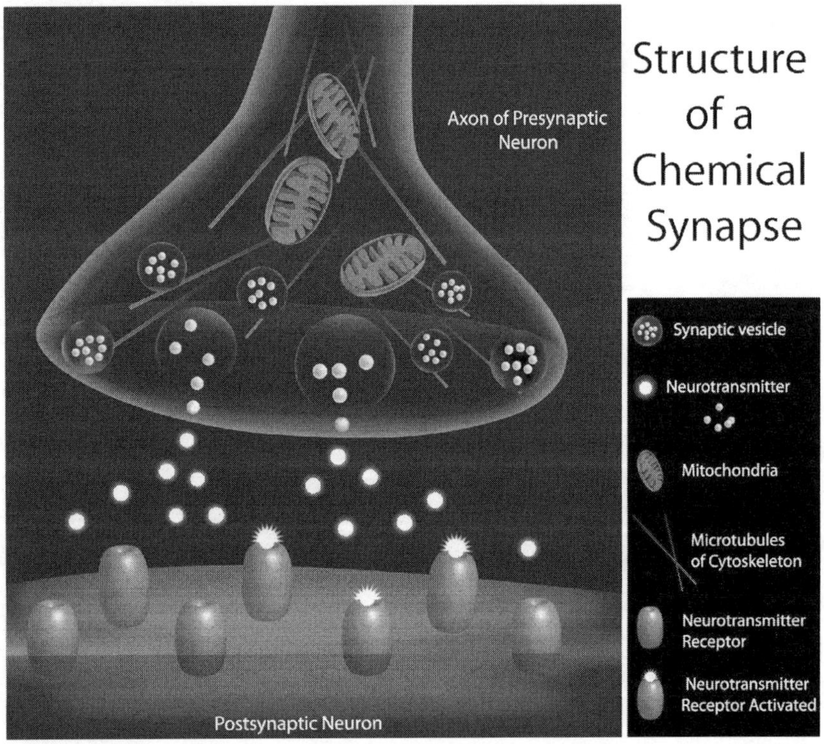

Figure 5.2
Synaptic cleft with acetylcholine and after acetylcholine esterase

light can activate again. But pesticides—specifically acetylcholine esterase inhibitors—disable the red light so that the insect is able to inhale while its heart is locked in a state of contraction. Sounds like a horrible way to die. But hey, no big deal right? After all, it's just a bug.

Well, what if I told you that your Nervous System is virtually identical to the insect's Nervous System? Your body uses acetylcholine as its major neurotransmitter, and acetylcholine esterase as its red light too. Chemical pesticides kill the bug, and then they have the exact same effect on your lungs, heart, and Nervous System once you eat the polluted produce. Still no big deal? Probably not.

Understand that acetylcholine and acetylcholine esterase are primarily responsible for the speed and recall accuracy of your memory, as well as the speed of your reflexes. Eating pollution disrupts this process, which has a adverse effect on your thought processes, decision-making, and ability to respond in ways that cultivate energy in your life.

Let's take a quick look again at how Americans die each year—Heart Disease, Cancer, Stroke, Chronic Lung Disease. Still think that conventionally grown produce is healthy for you? And what about the children? Pesticides have been linked to childhood asthma, ADD/ADHD, and lapses in concentration associated with poor performance in school. The smarter we are, the healthier we can be, the healthier we are, the more money we can save. Shouldn't we begin utilizing this concept to protect our children's health?

So are pesticides stressful to your body? Yes. They breakdown the Electron Transport Chain in your Mitochondria, create an acidic cellular environment, and disrupt your Nervous System, heart, and lungs. Because of this extraordinary level of stress, they also become a significant factor in the development most cancers.

The secret that Organic foods are better has been known since the time of Hippocrates. In his time, there was no distinction between conventional foods and Organic foods because there was no need—everything was Organic. The word Organic didn't exist because it didn't need to exist.

It is no accident that Organic foods have a higher concentration of nutrients than conventionally grown pesticide food. Doesn't the word "pesticide" just sound like a bad word? What you have to understand is that pesticides taint the where that foods are grown. Because pesticides also saturate the soil, they and their metabolites compete for absorption into the growing fruit, vegetable, grain, or legume. It's not enough to think that you can simply wash them off because, in reality, the act of washing pesticides from the surface of a food is less than 30 percent effective for the pesticides that are found on the outside of produce. *The only way to ensure that you are not ingesting pesticides is to make sure they are not in your diet.*

Every year, the Environmental Working Group (www.ewg.org) produces a wonderful guide about pesticides in produce called the *Dirty Dozen*. In their publication, they list the produce with the highest residue of pesticides. As a result, these food should be purchased Organically. I also want to stress that it is SOOOO much easier to buy all Organic produce than it is to shop in hopes of saving a few cents per pound. In fact, I will make an argument that it's actually a couple of dollars cheaper each month to shop Organic than it is to shop conventionally when you consider nutrient density.

Most Recent Dirty Dozen courtesy of EWG.org

1. Peaches	7. Strawberries
2. Apples	8. Kale
3. Bell Peppers	9. Lettuce
4. Celery	10. Imported Grapes
5. Nectarines	11. Carrots
6. Cherries	12. Pears

As a final thought of extreme importance about pesticides—understand that all pesticides are fat soluble. This means that they have an affinity for nervous tissue because it is surrounded by fat. Pesticides also have an affinity for your Lymphatic Chain where your Immune System resides, as well as your adipose tissue—otherwise known as your fat cells. Translation: Pesticides disrupt your Nervous System, heart, lungs, and Immune System, and they can be trapped in your body for decades—particularly if you are overweight or obese.

So eating Organic foods helps to reduce the stressful damage that pesticides wreak upon your Mitochondria. As a result, Organic foods can immediately benefit your health. Organic foods also are much higher in nutrient density than conventionally grown produce. Nutrient density is a new way of looking at food that enables you to compare the actual cost of conventionally grown foods and industrially produced foods with Organically grown and organically produced foods. It is no accident that despite the seemingly higher cost of Organic foods (which is a misnomer in itself), that the purchase of Organic foods has risen from 3 percent of all retail sales of produce in 2000, to more than 11 percent as of 2010 despite the economic recession. As a hopeful consequence of this rising trend in the demand for Organic foods, the total amount of farmland dedicated to Organic farming will grow beyond its current 1 percent allowance. It is also encouraging that consumer demand may very well inspire our government leaders to recognize the advantages of Organic foods, and begin to subsidize these foods and the companies that offer them. What a wonderful world we will make together!

Nutrient Density is defined as the amount of combined nutrients in a given food per calorie. Using this concept, let's take a conventionally grown peach at $1.50/pound, with a Nutrient Density of fifteen, and an unhealthy dose of pesticides, and compare it with an Organically grown peach at $2.00/pound, with a Nutrient Density of 150, and zero pesticides. The Organic peach will have significantly less pesticide residue than the conventionally grown peach. The Organic peach also will have a higher nutrient density than the conventionally grown peach. In addition, the initial cost per pound of the conventionally grown peach is less than the cost per pound of the Organically grown peach. It also is helpful to note that the *cost per nutrient-dense calorie* of the Organically grown peach ($0.013 per pound) is dramatically less than the cost per nutrient-dense calorie of the conventionally grown peach ($0.10 per pound). And finally, it will cost more to detoxify from the pesticides and preservatives in the conventionally grown peach than it will from the Organically grown peach. So with all of these factors considered, the conventionally grown peach costs more health-wise than the Organically grown peach.

So let's summarize the five arguments about the cost of Organic foods. First, they are absolutely affordable. Why not reallocate some of the 15 percent of the gross income that you spend on healthcare toward Eating Healthy? You'll feel better, and you will have more energy. You will turn your body into a detoxifying powerhouse, and you will SAVE A BUNCH OF MONEY in the process. How can you lose?

Five Truths of Organic Shopping

1. Zero Pesticide
2. Higher Nutrient Density
3. Illusion - Higher Cost per Pound
4. Reality – Lower Cost per Nutrient-Dense Calorie
5. Much Lower Cost to Detoxify Pesticides and Preservatives Compared to Conventional Foods

Additional Benefits of Organic Shopping

1. Higher Alkalinity and Energy Production
2. Lower Stress to Body and Mitochondria
3. Improved Clarity, Speed of Thought, and Reaction Times
4. Reduces Chemical Burden for Mother Earth
5. Develops Healthy, Smart Children
6. Saves Money and Trips to Doctor's Office
7. More Energy-Cultivating Responses

There is much more to talk about when it comes to Organic foods. And if I haven't convinced you by now, then you're just not going to change your mind. So I really hope that I've made a strong argument for Organic foods because they changed my life in the best way.

DELAYED FOOD ALLERGENS

While this is a topic we will discuss thoroughly in the chapter on the Immune System, it is important to make several points now. Delayed Food Allergies are one of the most underappreciated aspects of health in the medical field today. What if your Immune System had the responsibility of knowing which foods would be productive for your body, and which ones would not? Well, this is indeed the case. The only problem is that people are only tested for immediate reactions, and not delayed responses.

Immediate reactions to foods are reactions mediated through an **Immunoglobulin E** (IgE) antibody produced by cells from your Immune System. This reaction can begin within seconds, and symptoms can last from minutes up to several days. The half-life of this antibody in the bloodstream is approximately two days, which accounts for the relatively short duration of symptoms.

Delayed responses to foods are highly intelligent responses mediated through an **Immunoglobulin G** (IgG) antibody that is produced by cells in your Immune System. The IgG antibody is a much more sturdy class of antibody when compared to the IgE antibody. As a result, its effects have a much longer half-life (See **Figure 5.3**). The half-life of the IgG antibody is approximately twenty-one to twenty-eight days. A half-life is quite simple. It's the amount of time that it takes half of a substance to be reduced in your bloodstream. So as you can see, the IgG response is much longer than the IgE reaction to foods, and as a result, it is much more important to determine. Another characteristic of the IgG delayed response is that it will not begin until two hours or two days following exposure to an offending food. This can make it nearly impossible to isolate reactions simply through an elimination or rotation diet program. Fortunately, it can be tested for using a reputable lab and a simple blood draw. These can take all the guesswork out of your diet. The key here is the lab. A large number of labs test for delayed food allergies, but not all of them do it well. A good Naturopathic Doctor will help you sort through the list of viable options.

So, understanding which foods your Immune System likes and which it does not plays an essential role in Eating Healthy. If you are eating foods that your Immune System does not like, at least two things will work against you. First, any food that you have a delayed allergy to is immediately acidic

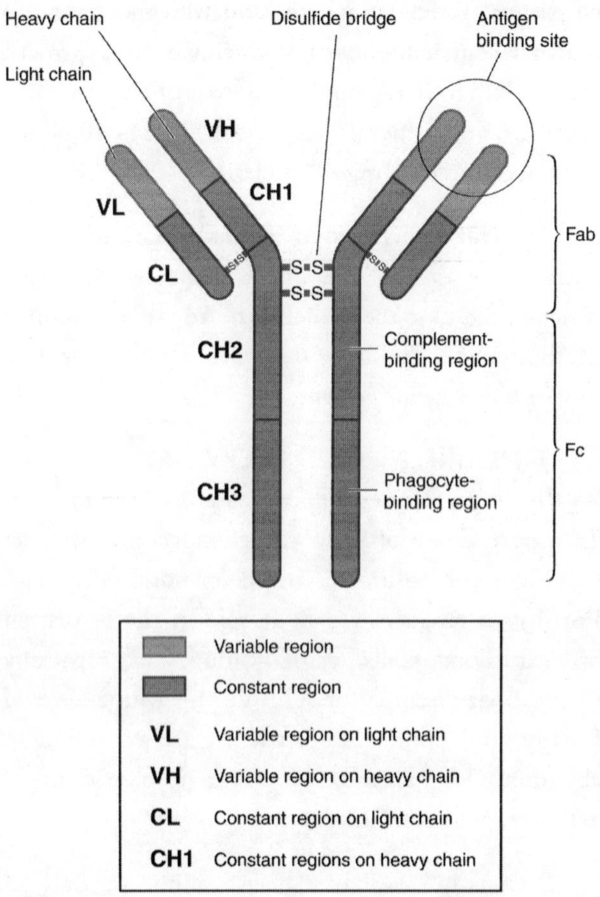

Figure 5.3
Notice the Antigen Binding Site. This is the location where the antibody effectively 'sticks' to whatever has been identified by Plasma Cells (B-Cells) as 'Not Self' so as to weigh the antigen down for other immune cells to scope it up and eat it (phagocytosis).

to your body, and it will create an acidic cellular environment, leading to damage and lower energy production. Second, any food that causes you to have a delayed allergy, will force your Immune System to attack it. As a result, your body will waste energy, and it will divert your Immune System away from handling its other responsibilities (e.g. killing infections, removing environmental pollution from your body). Eating foods that cause your body to mount immune responses, sets the stage for eventual immune-suppression. It also can turn you into a Bio-accumulating Organism.

SIXTY PERCENT ALKALIZING OR HIGHER

Years ago when I first started eating Organic, I conducted an experiment using Granny Smith Apples. I purchased one that was Organically grown, and one that was conventionally grown. Then I positioned both of them on a windowsill open to fresh air, but away from direct sunlight. Within three to four days, the Organic Granny Smith began to rot, but the conventionally grown one still looked as good as the day I bought it shiny and all. After a week, I had to throw the Organic apple away because it looked and began to smell pretty bad, but there still was no change in the conventional apple.

A month went by—no change.

Another month went by—no change.

Another month went by, and my friends began to ask me what I was doing. And still no change.

Another month went by, and I broke up with a girlfriend. Still no change.

A couple of months went by and there was no change.

Another month went by, and I found a new girlfriend. Still no change.

A couple of more months—no change.

Exactly one year later—no change.

So I thought to myself, *maybe it's been bad on the inside this whole time.* I cut it open and couldn't believe my eyes. It looked like an apple. Juice even came out. I called my ex-girlfriend to tell her, but she was not impressed. Oh well. A one-year-old apple that is still juicy is not a good thing. What was keeping this thing 'fresh?' Preservatives similar to embalming fluid. Is it possible that those same preservatives will start preserving your body? Yes, it is. For me, I'll take the apple, but the pesticides and preservatives? Forget it. That experiment sold me on Organic foods for life.

In chapter 3, we discussed pH, so let's do a little refresher here and consider the foods we eat. If you'll recall, a pH between 0 and 6.99 is acidic, a pH of 7.00 is neutral, and a pH of 7.01 to 14 is alkalizing. A discussion of foods and pH brings us to the **Principle of Advanced Natural Medicine #11**: *The pH of a food is determined by what effect it has on pH inside of the body, not by its pH outside the body. Enzymes, nutrients, antioxidants, and the energy of the food will have a direct influence on the pH of the body, and can be reasonably measured using urinary and salivary pH testing methods.*

Any food you eat that contains environmental pollutants like pesticides, preservatives, hormones, genetically modified organisms (GMOs), Polychlorinated biphenyl PCBs, plastics, antibiotics, MTBE, heavy metals, or other chemicals will be acidic to your body regardless of how alkalizing the food. Environmental pollution is enough to tip the balance into a noticeably acidic state.

Any food you eat that causes an IgE immune reaction or an IgG immune response will be acidic to your body regardless of how alkalizing it might have been to someone else. Remember that acid always leads to cellular damage, and it is an undeniable stressor.

Because of these realities, we strive for a meal that is at least 60 percent alkalizing when Eating Healthy. What this means is that 60 percent or more of what you eat in a meal directly contributes to alkalinity in your body. At the end of this chapter, I will provide an example that will show you how to calculate the alkalizing percentage using an alkalizing versus acidifying food and lifestyle chart I have supplied (See **Figure 5.4**) that shows which foods are alkalizing, and which ones are acidifying. You will see that various nutrition authors will have some information that is different than mine—which is fine. My chart is a summary of the latest research from my own clinical experience, my research of foods, and a long list of resources you can peruse in the citations. My chart also is heavily influenced by ORAC antioxidant capacity, and I will make a point that there is a direct correlation between Organic foods, nutrient density, antioxidant capacity, and alkalinity. Foods that are Organic and that are grown on nutrient-dense soils during optimal growth seasons will have the highest content of antioxidants, vitamins, and minerals. As a result, these will be the most alkaline forming of foods.

You will know a food is alkalizing and full of nutrients, enzymes, and antioxidants by the taste, which brings us to the **Principle of Advanced Natural Medicine #12**: *The better the flavor of a food, the more nutrients and Chi it possesses.*

EAT ONE GREEN FOOD EVERY DAY

In the previous chapter, we discussed the Electron Transport Chain of your Mitochondria and the fact that their composition is based on porphyrin rings. **Porphyrin rings** play a huge role in the formation of Red Blood Cells, detoxification, and especially in the final assembly of ATP during Mitochondrial Energy Production. And just where are we to find an abundance of naturally occurring porphyrin rings? Yep. Green, Green Chlorophyll.

Personally, I have been quite partial to Chlorella for more than a decade as my source of daily chlorophyll. It is renowned for having the highest density of chlorophyll of any food source on the planet, and as a result, it offers the highest concentration of porphyrin rings. Because of this fact, it is an excellent food source that helps optimize the energy production process. Chlorella also is known to produce Vitamin A, B Complex, C, D, E, K, as well as several minerals, including Calcium, Magnesium, Iron, Zinc, Potassium, Sodium, and Zinc. When you also consider that Chlorella contains a full spectrum of essential amino acids, more than eighteen amino acids, and healthy essential fatty acids, it's not difficult to understand why it is classified as a Superfood. Unique to Chlorella in the family of superfoods is a nutrient property called Chlorella Growth Factor (CGF). CGF is a nucleopeptide phytonutrient known to help repair the DNA of cells, and the DNA of Mitochondria. So this little magical food has the ability to do a great deal for your body, and also for your energy production.

Also in the family of Superfoods are Spirulina, Blue Green Algae, Wheatgrass, and Barley Grass. All are wonderful ways to Eating Healthy, even if their chlorophyll density is not as rich as that of chlorophyll. You also will find sizeable amounts of chlorophyll in any dark green leafy vegetable like Spinach, Kale, Collard Greens, and others. So this brings me to the **Principle of Advanced Natural Medicine #13**: *Eat Something Green Every Day!* I feel like I've been waiting forever to get that one out. Whew.

ORAC ANTIOXIDANTS

ORAC stands for Oxygen Radical Absorbance Capacity, meaning the ability of phytonutrients within a food or herb to effectively sponge up free radicals. When stress leads to an acidic cellular environment, damage is the ultimate result, which in turn, leads to the formation of a large number of free radicals. The best analogy I've ever been able to come up with to describe this process is to picture some big magnetic sponges, pinballs and a house where everything is made of fragile glass. Imagine that you are standing inside of this glass house, and you throw a couple of pinballs in any direction. Not hard to imagine that something is going to break, right? Now imagine that every time one of the pinballs hits glass, it creates three new pinballs that start bouncing around, wreaking havoc in different directions. Every time a pinball hits glass it multiplies and launches the new pin balls. This is essentially what free radicals do within your body—damage creates more free radicals, and as a result, more damage at the cellular level.

Now imagine some big magnetic sponges inside the house. With each new magnetic sponge, the antioxidant capacity increases. This effectively sponges up all the pinballs and halts the damage so that the body can begin the inflammatory process of healing. Now imagine that the magnetic sponges are present ALL THE TIME so that those pesky pinballs have nowhere to go.

Food and herbs with a high ORAC value will have the greatest ability to act as magnetic sponges, and as a result, they will have the highest antioxidant potential. This brings us to **Principle of Advanced Natural Medicine #14**: *Antioxidants stop damage before it starts.* If you want to feel young and look vibrantly youthful, Eating Healthy with ORAC Antioxidants is definitely for you.

For reference, please refer to **Figures 5.5** and **5.6**. **Figure 5.5** is an ORAC Top 80, while **Figure 5.6** includes antioxidant definitions that will help you classify various major phytonutrients.

REFINED SUGAR

Did you know that the U.S. Department of Agriculture (www.USDA.gov) has estimated that as of 2010, Americans will require more than seventy-one pounds of refined cane and beet sugar for every man, woman, and child in the country each year (See **Figure 5.7**)? This number does not include high-fructose corn syrup, or other natural and synthetic sweeteners. Seventy-one pounds on average— we really, really like our food sweet don't we?

Well, let's begin with some historical references. In 1901—when we were the healthiest nation on Earth and spent less than 2 percent of our gross income on healthcare—the average American consumed less than nineteen pounds of refined sugar each year. A little over on hundred years later, Americans are consuming on *average* between 120 and 280 pounds of refined sugars and sweeteners annually, depending on the information source. That's at least ten pounds of refined carbohydrate every month.

So let me get this straight—in 1901 we eat under two pounds of refined sugar each month, and now we're eating least ten pounds a month? I wish this wasn't the case, but because of this fact, we are dead last among 195 nations in our overall health.

How did this happen? First of all, everything—including conventionally produced meats—has sugar in it. Second, everything was conveniently labeled in grams instead of teaspoons. If I told you to take 10 teaspoons of sugar, and dump it in 12 ounces of water and gulp it down, you'd probably be repulsed. But that's exactly what you're doing every time you drink a can of soda or energy drink. Both are literally death in a can. So let me take them to task as a staple beverage of your diet. Do you like baseball?

Figure 5.4

Alkalizing vs. Acidifying Foods and Lifestyle

(+4) Most Alkalizing	(+3) More Alkalizing	(+2) Alkalizing	(+1) Least Alkalizing	Category
Loving, Satisfied, Joyful, Enthusiastic, Authentic	Patient, Peaceful, Confident, Truthful, Encouraging	Trusting, Faithful, Passionate, Calm	Rational, Tolerant	**Perspectives/ Emotional State**
Active 5X/Week	Active 4X/Week	Active 3X/Week	Active 2X/Week	**Exercise**
Eat at Home with Family 5X per week	Eat at Home with Family 4x per week	Eat at Home with Family 3x per week	Eat at Home with Family 1 – 2x per week	**Lifestyle**
8+ Hours Uninterrupted	8 Hours Uninterrupted	7.5 Hours Uninterrupted	7 Hours Uninterrupted	**Sleep**
Breathing Practice 60+ min/day	Breathing Practice 45 min/day	Breathing Practice 30 min/day	Breathing Practice 15 min/day	**Blood Gases**
Cloves, Cinnamon Oregano, Basil Turmeric Parsley	Thyme Cumin	Green Tea Ginger Peppermint, Spearmint Marjoram	Curry Sage Licorice Root Burdock Root	**Herbs**
Avocado Persimmon Papayas Lemons, Limes Blueberries	Plums BlackBerries Oranges, Tangelos Mango Grapes with Seeds	Apple, Pear Pineapple Raspberries Strawberries Peach Kiwi	Apricot, Nectarine Honeydew, Cantaloupe Banana Currant, Cherries Cooked Tomatoes Watermelon	**Fruits**
Spinach, Kale, Collards Swiss Chard, Greens Broccoli, Arugula Nori, Wakame, Kombu Hijiki	Cucumber, Zucchini Parsnip Green Leaf, Romaine Brussels Sprouts Boy Choy Fermented Soy	Sweet Potato Beets, Cauliflower Carrots Bell Peppers Pumpkin & Squash Garlic, Onions	Soy Beans, Tofu Jicama, Celery Green Peas, Asparagus Adzuki Beans, Black Beans Kidney Beans, Green Beans Hummus	**Vegetables & Legumes**
Wheat Grass Chlorella, Spirulina Blue - Green Algae Miso Soup	Most Vegetable Based Soups	Oats Sumac Sorghum Lentils	Quinoa Millet Amaranth	**Grains, Cereals, Grass, Soups**
Sprouts	Walnuts Pecans	Almonds Pistachio Hazelnut	Pumpkin Seeds Brazil Nuts Shitake	**Sprouts, Nuts, Mushrooms & Seeds**
	Cod Liver Oil	Evening Primrose Oil Borage Oil Cold Pressed Extra Virgin Olive Oil Flax Seed Oil	Avocado Oil Coconut Oil	**Oils**
			Perhaps Sushi If it is Wild Caught	**Meat Fowl Wild Game Shellfish**
	Breast Milk	Oat Milk Hemp Milk Almond Milk	Coconut Milk Rice Milk Soy Milk	**Dairy & Alternative Milks**
Herbal Organic Teas Ginseng Bicarbonate	High Quality Waters* Mineral Water	Sake with Miso Espresso Coffee	Filtered Water Honey Wine Red Wine	**Beverages**
Sea Salt		Black Strap Molasses Apple Cider Vinegar Umeboshi Stevia	Maple Syrup Raw Honey Raw Agave Rice Syrup	**Sweeteners Seasonings**
		Broad Spectrum Probiotics	Multivitamins, Antioxidants	**Extra**
				Totals

Reference 1. Prior, Wu. 'Oxygen Radical Absorbance Capacity of Selected Foods- 2007'. (Based on 20 References) 2. Mateljan. 'The World's Healthiest Foods' 2007. (based on 150+ References)

Category	(-1) Least Acidifying	(-2) Acidifying	(-3) More Acidifying	(-4) Most Acidifying
Perspectives/ Emotional State	Indifferent, Indecisive	Distrustful, Afraid, Lonely, Doubtful	Angry, Complaining, Frustrated, Isolated	Judgmental, Repressed, Controlling
Exercise	Active Without Sweating	Sedentary	Sedentary With Fast Food Diet	Sedentary + Fast Food + Sugar/Alcohol
Lifestyle	Eat Fast Food 1 – 2x per week	Eat Fast Food 3x per week	Eat Fast Food 4x per week	Eat Fast Food 5x per week
Sleep	6 Hours Uninterrupted	6 - 7 Hours Interrupted	5-6 Hours Interrupted	Less Than 5 Hours Total
Blood Gases	Shallow Breather	Shallow Breather w/ Kyphosis	Snore While Sleeping	Diagnosed with Sleep Apnea
Herbs				
Fruits	Sour Cherries Rhubarb Prune Raisin Dates	Cranberries Raw Tomatoes	Canned Fruit Shelf Juices w/ Sugar/Corn Syrup	All Non-Organic Fruit
Vegetables & Legumes	Potatoes String Beans Chick Peas	White Beans Navy Beans Pinto Beans	Processed Soy Products	All Non-Organic Vegetables
	Note: When Presoaked, Sprouted Beans Become More Alkalizing – Dr. Michio Kushi			
Grains, Cereals, Grass, Soups	Brown Rice Kasha Teff	Buckwheat Wheat Semolina Farina Spelt	Maize Corn Rye Barley White Rice	White Bread
Sprouts, Nuts, Mushrooms & Seeds	Peanuts Pine nuts Sunflower Seeds	Cashews		
Oils	Sesame Oil Grape Seed Oil Sunflower Oil Almond Oil Peanut Oil	Safflower Oil		Fried Foods Trans Fatty Acids Partially Hydrogenated Oils Crisco
Meat Fowl Wild Game Shellfish	**All Organic Free Range Meats & Eggs Pacific Wild Caught Fish**	Goat, Lamb Goose Turkey Shrimp Duck, Venison	Chicken Beef Eggs Crab, Scallops	Pork Oysters Lobsters Cat Fish Atlantic/Farmed Fish
Dairy & Alternative Milks	Goat cheese Sheep cheese Yogurt Goat Products	Aged Cheese Organic Dairy Products	Casein	Cheese Cow Milk Ice Cream Pus Cells
Beverages	Black Tea Sake	Lipton Tea	I Drink___Cups of Coffee per day	I Drink___Sodas, Diet Sodas, Alcoholic Beverages per day
Sweeteners Seasonings	Processed Honey Raw Sugar Brown Sugar	Vanilla	White Sugar Jams/Jellies Yeast	NutraSweet Equal Sweet n Low Splenda High Fructose Corn Syrup
Extra	L. Acidophilus			Antibiotics
Totals				

Figure 5.5

Antioxidant Rankings Top 80 and Notables

Top 1-40			Top 41-80		
Rank	ORAC Ranking	Total Antioxidant Capacity/100g serving	Rank	ORAC Ranking	Total Antioxidant Capacity/100g serving
1	**Cloves**	314446	41	**Black Beans**	8040
2	**Sumac Bran**	312400	42	**Pistachios**	7983
3	**Cinnamon**	267536	43	**Currants**	7960
4	**Oregano**	200129	44	**Blackberries**	7701
5	**Turmeric**	159227	45	**Plums**	7581
6	**Black Sorghum Bran**	100800	46	**Lentils**	7282
7	**Sumac Grain**	86800	47	**Dried Agave**	7274
8	**Cocoa**	80933	48	**Dried Apples**	6681
9	**Cumin**	76800	49	**Garlic Powder**	6665
10	**Parsley**	74349	50	**Raspberries**	6058
11	**Basil**	67553	51	**Lemon Balm**	5997
12	**Baking Chocolate**	49926	52	**Soy Beans**	5764
13	**Curry**	48504	53	**Garlic**	5346
14	**Sage**	32004	54	**Red Wine**	5034
15	**Mustard Seed**	29257	55	**Unpeeled Russet Potatos**	4882
16	**Ginger**	28811	56	**Sweet Cherries**	4873
17	**Black Pepper**	27618	57	**Basil**	4805
18	**Thyme**	27426	58	**Almonds**	4454
19	**Majoram**	27297	59	**Red Delicious Apples**	4275
20	**Rice Bran**	24287	60	**Raisins**	4188
21	**Chili Powder**	23636	61	**Granny Smith Apples**	3898
22	**Black Sorghum Grain**	21900	62	**Dates**	3895
23	**Dark Chocolate**	20823	63	**Walnuts**	3846
24	**Pecans**	17940	64	**Strawberries**	3577
25	**Paprika**	17919	65	**Dried Apricots**	3234
26	**Chokeberry**	16062	66	**Peanuts**	3166
27	**Tarragon**	15542	67	**Broccoli**	3083
28	**Ginger**	14840	68	**Raw Pears**	2941
29	**Elderberry**	14697	69	**Gala Apples**	2828
30	**Peppermint**	13978	70	**Cardamom**	2764
31	**Oregano**	13970	71	**Fuji Apples**	2589
32	**Small Red Beans**	13727	72	**Guava**	2550
33	**Wild Blueberries**	13427	73	**Oats**	2308
34	**Red Kidney Beans**	13259	74	**Raw Asparagus**	2150
35	**Pinto Beans**	11864	75	**Avocados**	1933
36	**Hazelnuts**	9645	76	**Oranges**	1819
37	**Cranberries**	9584	77	**Baked Potatoes**	1680
38	**Dried Pears**	9496	78	**Spinach**	1515
39	**Steamed Artichokes**	9416	79	**Sprouted Alfalfa Seeds**	1510
40	**Cultivated Blueberries**	9019	80	**Green Leaf Lettuce**	1447

Top Notables		
Rank	ORAC Ranking	Total Antioxidant Capacity/100g serving
	Herbs	
1	**Cloves**	314446
2	**Cinnamon**	267536
3	**Oregano**	200129
4	**Turmeric**	159227
5	**Cocoa**	80933
6	**Cumin**	76800
7	**Parsley**	74349
8	**Basil**	67553
9	**Baking Chocolate**	49926
10	**Curry**	48504
11	**Sage**	32004
12	**Ginger**	28811
Bonus	**Thyme**	27426
	Grains	
Higest	**Sumac Bran**	312400
	Black Sorghum Bran	100800
	Sumac Grain	86800
	Rice Bran	24287
Common	**Oats**	2308
	Wheat	1421
	Corn	728
	Nuts	
1	**Pecans**	17940
2	**Hazelnuts**	9645
3	**Pistachios**	7983
4	**Almonds**	4454
5	**Walnuts**	3846
	Beans & Legumes	
1	**Small Red Beans**	13727
2	**Red Kidney Beans**	13259
3	**Pinto Beans**	11864
	Produce	
1	**Wild Blueberries**	13427
2	**Cranberries**	9584
3	**Steamed Artichokes**	9416
4	**Blackberries**	7701
5	**Plums**	7581
6	**Raspberries**	6058
7	**Sweet Cherries**	4873

Figure 5.6

MAJOR ANTIOXIDANTS DEFINITIONS

Class	Forms & Names	Function	Awesome Sources
Carotenoids	Vitamin A, Beta Carotene, Lycopene	Promotes Optimal Functioning of the Immune System. Improves Vision. Necessary for Bone growth & development. Essential for the replication of epithelial cells (Skin, Intestines, Lungs) during wound healing.	Chlorella, Spirulina, Carrots, Sweet Potatoes, Kale, Parsley, Spinach, Watercress, Raw Carrots, Cooked Tomatoes, Mangos, Pumpkins, Squash
Ascorbic Acid	Vitamin C, Mineral Ascorbate, Buffered	Antioxidant. Aids in Iron absorption. Necessary for specific hormone and neurotransmitter synthesis. Liver Detoxification. Lowers Cholesterol.	Camu-Camu Berries, Acerola berries, Oranges, Guava, Green Peppers, Grapefruit
D-Tocopherol	Vitamin E	Antioxidant. Protects cell membranes, especially Red Blood Cells & Lungs. Vital for Nerve and Muscle Cell activity. Anti-inflammatory.	Wheat Germ, Sunflower Seeds, Almonds, Pecans
Polyphenols	Phenols, Phenolic Acids, Indole-3-Carbonol	Produced by plants to offset infection antioxidants in this class offer anti-inflammatory properties as well as anti-viral in some cases.	Green Tea, Nettle Root, Peppermint, Spearmint, Lemon Balm, Blueberry, Hawthorn Berry, Blackberry
Flavonoids	Bioflavonoids, Isoflavones, Flavones, Catechins, Quercetin	Found widely in the plant world, over 4,000 different forms have been identified to date. A member of the Polyphenol family that impart color to fruits and flowers (orange, yellow, white). ***Essential for a healthy cardiovascular system.***	Green Tea, Artichokes, Asparagus, Celery, Chives, Pears, White Eggplant, Citrus Fruits (Fibers Between Fruit & Rind), Soy Beans, Red Kidney Beans
Anthocyanins	Proanthocyanins, Oligoprocyanins(OPCs)	Another special member of the Polyphenol family that impart color to fruits and flowers, typically blues, purples, and reds. ***Essential for a healthy cardiovascular system.***	Blueberries, Blackberries, Hawthorn Berries, Pine Bark, Red Grape Seeds
Various Antioxidants	Co-Q-10, Glutathione, N-Acetyl Cysteine, Alpha Lipoic Acid	Essential co-factors in energy production, antioxidant & enzyme production within the body, and/or free-radical absorption.	Wide Assortment of Legumes, Grains, Vegetables, & Herbs
Fish Oils	EPA (Eicosapentaenoic Acid), DHA (Docosahexaenoic Acid)	Neuroprotective Antioxidants essential for proper neural development in children.	Cod Liver Oil, Krill Oil
Antioxidants	Longevity, Anti-aging, Nature's Little Miracles	That which provides longevity by absorbing free radicals produced from stress. Antioxidants are especially essential in wound & tissue healing, maintaining a healthy cardiovascular system, and limiting damage from Auto-immune diseases.	Colorful Fruits & Vegetables, Legumes, Grains, Red Wine, Dark Beers, and especially concentrated in Herbs.
Free Radicals	Reactive Oxygen Species (ROS), Superoxide, Peroxyl Radicals, Hydroxyl Radicals, Peroxynitrite	Substances formed from Acidic pH, Inflammation, Immune Reactions, Cellular Metabolism, and the Stresses of Life. These substances act to destroy cell structures.	Emotional Stress, Dietary Stress, Poor Biomechanical Alignment, Scar Tissue, all of which lead people into Acidic Cellular Environments.
Antioxidant Measurement Techniques	ORAC (Oxygen Radical Absorbance Capacity) FRAP (Ferric Reducing Antioxidant Power) TRAP (Total Radical-Trapping Antioxidant Parameter) TEAC (Trolox Equivalent Antioxidant Capacity)	In vitro methods to assess for antioxidant capabilities in foods.	See References

Figure 5.7

Table 26
U.S. sugar long-term projections

Item	Units	2008/09	2009/10	2010/11	2011/12	2C12/13	2013/14	2014/15	2015/16	2016/17	2017/18	2018/19	2019/20
Sugarbeets													
Planted area	1,000 acres	1,091	1,173	1,182	1,154	1,140	1,144	1,142	1,140	1,137	1,134	1,132	1,132
Harvested area	1,000 acres	1,005	1,156	1,133	1,105	1,092	1,096	1,093	1,091	1,088	1,086	1,085	1,084
Yield	Tons/acre	26.8	25.5	26	25.9	25.9	26	26.1	26.2	26.3	26.4	26.5	26.6
Production	Mil. s. tons	27	29.5	29.4	28.6	28.3	28.5	28.6	28.6	28.7	28.7	28.8	28.8
Sugarcane													
Harvested area	1,000 acres	824	809	801	797	798	799	800	802	803	803	801	791
Yield	Tons/acre	32.2	33.6	34.1	34	34.2	34.4	34.6	34.7	34.9	35.1	35.3	35.5
Production	Mil. s. tons	26.6	27.2	27.3	27.1	27.3	27.5	27.7	27.8	28	28.2	28.2	28.1
Supply:													
Beginning stocks	1,000 s. tons	1,660	1,451	1,016	1,473	1,496	1,503	1,513	1,522	1,531	1,539	1,548	1,555
Production	1,000 s. tons	7,484	7,713	7,741	7,649	7,647	7,714	7,759	7,803	7,843	7,884	7,918	7,930
Beet sugar	1,000 s. tons	4,166	4,400	4,477	4,396	4,371	4,412	4,430	4,448	4,463	4,482	4,500	4,525
Cane sugar	1,000 s. tons	3,318	3,313	3,264	3,253	3,276	3,302	3,329	3,355	3,380	3,403	3,417	3,405
Total Imports	1,000 s. tons	3,082	2,427	3,624	3,454	3,497	3,500	3,522	3,544	3,569	3,592	3,611	3,661
TRQ Imports	1,000 s. tons	1,370	1,257	1,309	1,311	1,317	1,319	1,322	1,324	1,329	1,332	1,334	1,337
Other imports	1,000 s. tons	1,712	1,170	2,315	2,143	2,181	2,181	2,200	2,220	2,240	2,260	2,276	2,323
Total supply	1,000 s. tons	12,226	11,591	12,382	12,576	12,640	12,718	12,793	12,868	12,943	13,016	13,076	13,146
Use:													
Exports	1,000 s. tons	137	200	200	200	200	200	200	200	200	200	200	200
Domestic deliveries	1,000 s. tons	10,638	10,375	10,709	10,880	10,937	11,005	11,071	11,138	11,203	11,268	11,321	11,382
Miscellaneous	1,000 s. tons	0	0	0	0	0	0	0	0	0	0	0	0
Total use	1,000 s. tons	10,774	10,575	10,909	11,080	11,137	11,205	11,271	11,338	11,403	11,468	11,521	11,582
Total Pounds		21,548,000,000	21,150,000,000	21,818,000,000	22,160,000,000	22,274,000,000	22,410,000,000	22,542,000,000	22,676,000,000	22,806,000,000	22,936,000,000	23,042,000,000	23,164,000,000
Pounds Per American				71									
CCC surplus disbursements 1/	1,000 s. tons	0	0	0	0	0	0	0	0	0	0	0	0
Ending stocks	1,000 s. tons	1,451	1,016	1,473	1,496	1,503	1,513	1,522	1,531	1,539	1,548	1,555	1,564
Raw sugar price:													
New York, No. 16 contract	Cents/lb.	26.04	24.98	22.92	22.92	22.92	22.92	22.92	22.92	22.92	22.92	22.92	22.92
Raw sugar loan rate	Cents/lb.	18	18.25	18.5	18.75	18.75	18.75	18.75	18.75	18.75	18.75	18.75	18.75
Beet sugar loan rate	Cents/lb.	23.13	23.45	23.77	24.09	24.09	24.09	24.09	24.09	24.09	24.09	24.09	24.09
Grower prices:													
Sugarbeets	Dol./ton	45	43.58	40.66	39.47	39.47	39.47	39.47	39.47	39.47	39.47	39.47	39.47
Sugarcane	Dol./ton	28.7	29.05	28.63	28.92	29.37	29.81	30.26	30.7	31.15	31.6	32.03	32.42

This means that there is 71 pounds of sugar available for every man, woman and child in 2010
So it is not far-fetched to think that the average American consumes between 150 and 300 pounds annually
since this number does not include HFCS or any other refinement of sugar.

Note: Marketing year beginning October 1 for sugar.
1/ CCC is the Commodity Credit Corporation, U.S. Department of Agriculture.

Soda is one of the most acidic substances you can put in your body. The average 12-ounce can of soda has about 40 grams of refined sugar in it—**STRIKE 1!** What the heck is a gram? That's what I used to think. I know what a teaspoon is, a cup is, a gallon is. If someone told you one of those units of measurement you could probably conceptualize it—but a gram? They might as well have used a hammock of cake as a unit of measurement, because it's just as meaningless.

So let me explain what this means. *ONE TEASPOON OF SUGAR IS EQUAL TO 4 GRAMS.* So, when you read a label that has refined sugar in it, you can safely estimate the number of teaspoons of sugar by dividing the number of grams by 4. For example, a 12-ounce soda has 40 grams of sugar in it. So if you divide 40 by 4, you will discover that there are 10 teaspoons of sugar in that beverage. And we wonder why our children bounce off of walls and won't pay attention to us after a sugar rush? Your body only needs 1 teaspoon of sugar floating in the bloodstream to function at an optimal level.

Soda also is made from filtered tap water that is full of heavy metals, chlorine, chloroform, fluoride, germs, antibiotics, antidepressants, MTBE (that's rocket fuel), and plastics. The filtered tap water also is usually from a reclaimed or treated source, meaning that it's recycled from your bathroom toilet. Yes, it is that gross, and it's also...**STRIKE 2!**

Most sodas also are carbonated, which means that carbon dioxide is pumped into the water to give it that fizzy, bubbly, effervescence. Well, the problem with this is that carbon dioxide is the very gas we are trying to get rid of every time we exhale because it is highly acidic...**STRIKE 3!**

Sodas also typically come in a can or plastic bottle, but due to the acidic pH, there is the unique opportunity for a mass transfer of either aluminum or phthalate (plastic) into the beverage...**STRIKE 4!**

But before you start thinking that you'll switch to diet soda, think again. And don't even get me started on the effects of artificial sweeteners on neurotransmitters and the Immune System.

It is important for you to understand some key information about your body. *Your body functions optimally well with a blood sugar level that is equivalent to 1 teaspoon of sugar.* That's right—all your body needs to perform very, very well is 1 teaspoon of sugar distributed throughout its 5 liters of blood. So when you drink a beverage or eat a food with a large amount of sugar, you are creating a highly acidic environment in your bloodstream and effectively throwing off the pH levels throughout your body. With every 12 ounces of soda you drink, you are ingesting ten times the amount of sugar that your body needs to function. And what will your cells do with the excess? They will store it as triglycerides in your fat. But let's say your body is tired of this daily overload you've been subjecting it too for a couple of years or more. What happens? Say hello to the most common cause of insulin resistance—known as Type II Diabetes. I'll never forget a ten-year-old child I had to diagnose with Type II Diabetes. Her mother felt helpless because she was unable to stop her ten-year-old from drinking 2 liters of soda every day after school. Let's just say that I gave that mom an education and a piece of my mind.

So what's the take-home message for you from this section? Remember that your body only needs 1 teaspoon of sugar to function properly. Know that you now have the power to convert grams of refined sugar into teaspoons so that you know what you are thinking about putting into your body. Know that soda should only be an occasional indulgence, and not a staple of Eating Healthy. Also know that agave sweetener and other natural sweeteners are not much better as sweeteners, except for the additional mineral they *might* provide. The best beverages have always been clean water, herbal teas, and fresh Organic juices.

Let me leave you with this final thought, and why I say Eating Healthy is no more than 8 grams or 2 teaspoons of refined sugar per major meal. In 1958, 1.58 million Americans were diagnosed with Diabetes. As of 2008, there were 23.6 million Americans diagnosed with Diabetes, not counting the additional 6 million were not yet diagnosed. Not coincidentally, the annual consumption of refined sugar and sweeteners continues to increase every year. Diabetes also happens to be a major factor in the development of Heart and Cardiovascular Disease—the leading cause of death in the United States. So, let's throw in the **Principle of Advanced Natural Medicine #15**: *If it walks like a duck and talks like a duck...it's a duck.*

NATURALLY SWEET

Eating something naturally sweet is important. A sweet flavor helps stimulate either Energy-Cultivating Responses or Energy-Draining Reactions. If a food or beverage contains concentrated refined sugars, then the result is a stressful acidic cellular environment, damaging, free radicals, and Energy-Draining Reactions. These Energy-Draining Reactions include—but are not limited to—excessive mental chatter and the feeling of becoming easily overwhelmed. Imagine that you just drank a soda to satisfy your craving for something sweet. You overwhelm your bloodstream with sugar. Is it possible that you will begin to feel overwhelmed by life? Excessive use of refined sugar also can exacerbate insomnia and TMJ Syndrome, depending on how the high load of sugar adversely impacts the Nervous System.

By contrast, eating something sweet—in a natural form that promotes an Alkaline Cellular Environment—promotes Mitochondrial Energy Production, detoxification, and Energy-Cultivating Responses. Refer to the Genesis Energetics—5-Element Perspective (See **Figure 2.2**) for a moment. When the body craves something sweet, it is attempting to stimulate Energy-Cultivating Responses. Your body is not designed to desire the production of energy draining experiences, because to do so would be in direct opposition to its innate tendency to promote life. So, alkalizing foods that also are naturally sweet stimulate rational decision-making, along with clear and calm mental states. The sweet flavor produces energy and works to aid the decision-making process, which builds positive momentum in your life. *Your body wants to help you make your dreams come true.* In fact, it is designed to assist you in this life process.

The better you become at interpreting and acting on what your body is saying to you, the more adept you will become at making decisions that bring your dreams closer and closer to reality.

TOTAL FIBER

Fiber often is discussed in terms of how much you should eat every day. In fact, the current recommendations fall between 25 to 35 grams a day. Of course, this is based on three square meals each day, which I do not recommend adults eat unless they are very athletic and in need of a higher caloric intake to support the demands they are placing on their bodies. As part of a calorie-restricted practice, I recommend one major meal each day, one light meal, and several healthy alkalizing snacks. So, if we simply divide the current recommended daily intake by three, we come up with a very safe Eating Healthy Guideline of 8 to 12 grams per major meal.

Fiber does at least five beautiful things that we will discuss in more detail in Volume 2 and Volume 3 of this text. First of all, fiber acts as a bulking agent for your digestive tract. As a bulking agent, it gives the muscles of your digestive tract something significant to push against so that they can remain strong and toned. As with any muscle, use it or lose it. Secondly, fiber also acts to bind waste and excess hormones that are detoxified and released by your Liver. As a result, fiber is an essential part of any detoxification program. Fiber also creates a very gentle abrasive action, which helps clean your digestive tract, while promoting strong muscles along the way. It also has the ability to slow the absorption of nutrients into your bloodstream. This helps regulate healthy blood sugars, and can help the body tolerate high doses of nutrients. In fact, it is recommended that virtually all supplemental nutrients be taken with some form of natural fiber preceding them. And last of all, fiber breaks down into short chain fatty acids that help fuel the cells of the large intestine, helping to prevent atrophy and colon cancer. Every ounce of prevention is worth pounds of cure.

So to sum it up, 8-12 grams of fiber with every major meal helps optimize and regulate your digestion, blood sugars, the detoxification process, and ability to eliminate waste. No system of naturopathic principles should be without mention of bowel movements. **Principle of Advanced Natural Medicine #16**: *The number of poops per day should equal the number of major meals eaten per day. One poop per meal—that's the minimum.*

RAW FRUITS OR VEGETABLES

The main reason for including something raw in your meal is for the naturally occurring enzymes found within. You may be familiar with papain from raw papayas, or bromelain from the stems of pineapples as potent digestive aids. You also may be familiar with several other classes of enzymes, including proteases that assist in breaking down proteins and lipases that help breakdown fats. It is important to note that prolonged cooking methods have a tendency to destroy the enzyme potential of most foods.

Raw is often described as a living food because of the prevalence of naturally occurring enzymes, which have a positive impact on the health of your digestive system, joints, and thought processes. Similar to how antioxidants stop damage before it starts, enzymes in raw fruits and vegetables help breakdown foods and also spare your body from overexerting itself while digesting meals. It takes a tremendous amount of energy to breakdown, absorb, and eliminate a meal. Eating Organic, alkalizing raw foods can provide a tremendous assist to the digestive process, while helping your body conserve energy. Does everything need to be raw to be effective? At the risk of angering the raw community, my clinical opinion would have to be no. But, does raw food help make meals more digestible, and as a result, help you conserve your energy? There can be little argument about this fact.

The nice thing about enzymes is that they are similar to antioxidants in another way. Antioxidants stop damage before it starts, while enzymes found in raw fruits and vegetables have the ability to stop damage almost immediately after it starts—particularly in the joints. This makes eating raw foods a fantastic medicine for most arthritic conditions. Enzymes found in food serve a dual purpose in your body. On the one hand, they help you to digest the meal. On the other hand, they have the ability to interrupt the inflammatory process.

The significant fact to note about raw foods is the presence of a particular antioxidant called Quercetin. Quercetin is found in very high quantities in virtually all Organic fruits and vegetables, and it has some fantastic properties. First of all, Quercetin is best known to be a mast cell stabilizer, which means that it has a wonderful effect on allergies and sinus conditions—particularly when used in conjunction with Omega-3 Fatty Acids, which are typically found in Flaxseed and Fish Oils. Secondly, as we noted in chapter 4, Quercetin is responsible for making energy production much more efficient. But it is the third property that excites me the most because it is the least-known fact about the antioxidant. Quercetin speeds up the rate of nerve conduction, which allows your Nervous System to communicate faster. *This means that if you are a student or professional, it will help you think faster, and if you are an athlete or in the performing arts, it will improve your reaction times.*

Like enzymes, Quercetin is very unstable when exposed to heat at temperatures that are too high, or for prolonged periods of time. This is another good argument for Eating Healthy, and making a portion of your meal raw. A study I read in 2010 reported that in Organic foods, Quercetin can be found in concentrations that are up to four hundred times greater than those found in conventionally grown produce. This is another strong argument for Organic foods.

As a general rule, the longer you cook your food, the greater likelihood that enzyme content, antioxidants like Quercetin and other nutrients will be destroyed in the process. While this is true of most plant-based food sources, there are a few notable exceptions where heat is actually needed to liberate the antioxidant potential. In the category of

Healthy Oil Recommendations		
No Heat	Molecularly Distilled and Pollution-Free Fish Oil, Flaxseed Oil, Hemp Oil	All are good sources of healthy Omega-3 Fatty Acids
Low-Medium Heat	Olive Oil, Sesame	Light Sautéing, Sauces, Soups
Medium-High Heat	High-Oleic Sunflower Oil, Coconut Oil, Almond Oil, Peanut Oil	Baking, Frying, Searing, Browning, Deep Frying

better cooked than raw would be tomatoes for their Lycopene, artichokes, cabbage and potatoes. What's interesting is that this same study also demonstrated a clear antioxidant superiority for unpeeled fruits and vegetables over produce that had been peeled, which confirms what your grandmother probably told you: "Eat the peel… it's good for you."

HEALTHY PREPARATION METHODS

One of the coolest things I've learned comes from some of the resources listed at the end of this chapter. *The World's Healthiest Foods*, researched and authored by George Mateljan, is simply a work of mastery and an essential guide for nutrition. He does such a thorough and fantastic job of organizing and simplifying nutrition, AND showing you how easy it is to make healthy food taste incredible. Because of this, I have made his work required reading for all of my patients and students. He is a true inspiration.

One of the things that I learned early on is that we tend to overcook our food. In doing so, we destroy much of the nutrient density that we are paying top dollar for when we purchase Organic foods. In his book, George has an entire section titled, "Healthiest Way of Cooking" that is about as informative as any instruction guide on food preparation you will find. Without giving away too much—because I really want you to buy his book if you haven't already—I'll list some main ideas about healthy food preparation that I've developed, along with several of George's nifty concepts. Understand that his concepts on healthy preparation methods are revolutionary and rock solid. They are an example of Sophisticated Simplicity applied to daily life. I promise you that you will not be disappointed by his work. Thank You George.

Ideas for Healthy Preparation Methods When Cooking

1. Use Environmentally Safe Cookware.
2. Use lids to preserve nutrients that may be carried off by any steam leaving the cookware.
3. Cook at low to medium temperatures to maximize the retention of nutrients, and to make the meal easier to digest.
4. Cook for short periods of time using the methods for Healthy Sautéing, Healthy Steaming, Quick Broiling, and Quick Boiling as outlined by George Mateljan.
5. Use alternatives for Cow Milk, such as Rice, Oat, Coconut, Almond, Hemp, and Soy at every opportunity. Alternative milks can be safely used as a 1:1 replacement for Cow Milk with absolutely ZERO loss in taste.
6. Use distilled water for soups and herbal teas to maximize the extraction of nutrients into the water.
7. Use bottled spring water for all other cooking needs, including boiling, and steaming.
8. Use Celtic sea salt, Himalayan salt, or pink salt for seasoning over iodized salt. The additional trace minerals found in sea salt and pink salt help to better regulate blood pressure.

9. When using garlic, fresh-press each clove and add it to your food at the end of cooking. Pressing garlic activates a very amazing germ killer called Allicin, and as a result, it turns garlic from a seasoning into a medicine.

10. Use the right oil for the right temperature. I strongly recommend having three different oils in your kitchen—oils for no heat, low to medium heat, and medium to high heat.

And now a final recommendation on selecting healthy oils. Select Organic, cold pressed, and dark bottled whenever possible. Using an oil at a temperature in excess of its capacity leads to the formation of unhealthy trans-fatty acids. If the oil you are cooking with begins to smoke, allow it to cool and then dispose of it. Any oil that smokes has reached a temperature that is too high, and that has started to convert into an unhealthy trans-fatty acid. Any medium-high heat oil also can be used as a low-medium heat oil (see chart on previous page).

ENVIRONMENTALLY SAFE MEATS

Did you know that, according to the Union of Concerned Scientists, 70 percent of all antibiotics and related drugs are given to livestock?

We all seem to have this wonderful image of a peaceful farm, with the sun peeking through fluffy clouds, and the animals going about the business of whatever they do with their days on a peaceful farm. We envision cows grazing on wild grasses with their tails slowly shaking away the pester of flies. We think of little piglets rolling in the mud with a cartoon smile on their faces. We have a mental image of chickens walking freely around the yard, pecking away as a cat and dog lounge on the front porch. There's green everywhere, and in the background, are the fields of corn. This idyllic farm scene also includes the big red barn where the animals sleep until the morning, when a day in this simple life starts all over again.

The scene I just described might have been the norm in 1901, but certainly not in 1991. Today, virtually everything is conventionally grown, or industrialized. The conditions in which animals are raised is one step short of purposefully malicious. And shame on us for allowing an animal that's intended to give its life for our sustenance to have to live its life in such conditions. There is a major hypocrisy that perpetuates itself in our great nation, and it can be found in the way we treat our animals. If a person harms a dog or a cat, then they can be fined—or in extreme cases, lose their jobs or be sent to jail. But for animals intended for our consumption, we turn a blind eye to the vicious and horrific ways that they are raised and treated. No animal should have to live its entire life caged, beaten, and lying in its own excrement. After all, they're just food—they don't have any feelings, right? How does it make sense that a man can go to jail for killing dogs, but not be punished for mistreating an animal that is raised to help sustain our physical body?

Every time you spend a dollar on conventional industrial meat, you are supporting the way these animals are mistreated and brutally slaughtered. All of that waste that they sleep in, and all of the trauma they see, hear, and live each day of their miserable lives gets trapped in their tissue. And then we eat their flesh and can't seem to figure out why we feel so bad. Maybe we're feeling just a little of what they have felt. Maybe the disease we develop from eating these animals is repayment for their lifetime of mistreatment. If you think I'm making this up or exaggerating, by all means watch *Food, Inc.* and do your own research. It's enough to make vegetarianism look very, very attractive.

While I do enjoy vegetarian days, I also consume free-range and Organic meat. After years of teaching nutrition, I knew the living conditions that animals lived in on conventional, industrial farms, but I played this out-of-sight, out-of-mind game with myself. Because I didn't see the images, I could pretend they weren't happening—until I watched *Food, Inc.* After watching this courageous documentary and seeing how chickens live cramped and too heavy from the hormone to even walk, and how cows are pushed around by forklifts, and then to hear their screams and see the terror in their eyes—it finally all mattered to me. And it matters to me a great deal. After all, we're asking them to give up their lives for us. The least we can do is honor them and the sacrifice they are making for us with a good life, and a humane, peaceful death. It makes sense energetically to do so. It makes sense for us to do this for selfish reasons too. Don't you want the meat you eat to be clean? You see, *every dollar you spend is a vote cast.* One of my great hopes in life is to live to see the day when all fast-food companies begin to offer Organic free-range meats and produce. I dream of a day when we won't need to use the word "Organic" anymore, and when we can fully realize that a cow's life is every bit as important as a dog's life. Anything that will eventually become you should be clean and nutrient dense. Watch *Food, Inc.* Watch it, vote differently with your dollar, and let's find out what we can really do. *The best way to change government policy and industrial neglect isn't with petitions or marches. The best way to force change is with your wallet.*

So what's in all that government-subsidized, cheap, polluted, conventional industrial meat?

Did you know that peaceful farms have turned into polluted and infected Confined Animal Feeding Operations (CAFOs)?

Did you know that the cows, pigs, chickens, turkeys, and lambs on these CAFOs are fed more than 13.5 million pounds of antibiotics each year, plastic pellets for fiber, GMO grains, manure, animal excrement, and same-species meat from diseased animals that includes feathers, hair, Skin, and blood?

Did you know that a large percentage of cysts, pockets of infections, and diseased tissues are cut away before the food is packaged and shipped to the local supermarket?

Did you know that ground beef often is made up of tens, if not hundreds, of different cows?

Did you know that these animals develop disease from the filthy living conditions, lack of movement associated with being confined to a cage, and the stress of hearing other animals brutally slaughtered?

This is systematized insanity. There HAS to be a better way than this. How can we not see that an animal full of pollution and infections will lead to Acidic Cellular Environments in our own bodies, along with all the inevitable diseases that go along with those conditions? It is impossible to be healthy if conventional industrial meat is a staple of your diet—that is, unless someone figures out how to get healthy from eating infections, pus, and disease.

How we care for the animals that we end up eating is as big of a problem as pesticide-heavy produce and our excessive consumption of refined sugar when considering our physical and emotional health. Think back to 1901—were there any pesticides? Nope. Did we consume hundreds of pounds of sugar every day? Nope. Were there CAFOs? Nope. Was there an inordinate amount of money spent on healthcare and pharmaceuticals? Nope. Was there Fast-food? Nope. Was there a federal deficit? Nope. Were there billions of pounds of pollution produced every year? Nope.

Fortunately, there is a wonderful solution to this problem without going 100 percent vegetarian—even though going vegetarian can be a worthwhile solution to explore in and of itself. The solution is Organic and Free-Range Meats that are raised and Grass-Fed.

Shouldn't an animal—who has been designated from birth to give its life for a meal—be allowed to walk around and graze for a couple of hours each day? Is that too much to ask?

Did you know that Organic and Free-Range meats—meaning animals who are allowed to walk around and graze—are substantially more nutrient dense than those raised in conventional, industrial environments? Did you know that free-range and Organic meat tastes remarkably better? Did you know that the USDA and Clemson University did a comprehensive study in 2009 that came to the following conclusions:

USDA and Clemson Study on Grass-Fed vs. Grain-Fed Beef

1. Grass-fed beef is lower in total fat and saturated fats.

2. Grass-fed beef is higher in Vitamin A, Vitamin E, and Vitamin B-Complex.

3. Grass-fed beef is higher in calcium, magnesium, and potassium.
4. Grass-fed beef is higher in anti-inflammatory Omega-3 Essential Fatty Acids.
5. Grass-fed beef has a healthier ratio of Omega-3 to Omega-6 Essential Fatty Acids.
6. Grass-fed beef is higher in CLA, a cancer-fighting nutrient.
7. Grass-fed beef is lower in pro-inflammatory Arachidonic Acid.

If you are interested in how to make a positive change in the lives of farm animals, please purchase your meat and eggs that are free-range and Organic, and contact the Global Animal Partnership. The Global Animal Partnership is a multinational group that is dedicated to continually improving the lives of farm animals. Any farm that is rated 4+ or higher is a farm worth supporting because it is taking care of animals the right way, and delivering a much higher-quality product.

This brings us to the **Principle of Advanced Natural Medicine #17**: *If it's not Organic, it's not food.*

ENVIRONMENTALLY SAFE FISH

With farm-raised and lake-caught fish, there are three primary concerns regarding environmental pollution—Mercury, PCBs, and paint. Yes, I said paint. Imagine that you could select the color of the fish you eat, just like you choose the color of your kitchen walls. Well you don't have to imagine this, because it's already happening.

Did you know that farm-raised salmon gets its pink color from a chemical known as canthaxanthin? The chemical enables the farmer to choose what shade of pink he wants the flesh to be. That's right. Salmon fish farmers actually look through color swatches to determine what color they would like their fish to be, and canthaxanthin is then added to the fish feed. If the fish farmer omitted this step, farm-raised salmon would be a very unattractive, dull, and lifeless gray color. Did someone say YUCK?

The environmentally safest seafood is Alaskan Wild Caught. After a chapter this big, let's just keep this section simple—*Eating Alaskan Wild Caught Seafood = Eating Healthy.*

ENVIRONMENTALLY SAFE COOKWARE

Teflon Toxicosis. Teflon Toxicosis is a type of environmental pollution created by non-stick pans. It is created when the surface of a pan begins to disintegrate, creating known carcinogenic gases. A study conducted by the Environmental Working Group in 2003 reported that non-stick coating—under normal heating ranges—at least two carcinogens, two global pollutants, and a chemical that is lethal to humans at low doses. The study also reported that the non-stick surface breaks down at high temperatures, and turns into a nerve gas similar to one used during WWII. Think that might affect your mood and energy levels?

Below is a list of safe cookware. Notice how most of the cookware are items we've been using for hundreds, if not thousands, of years.

Environmentally Safe Cookware and Storage

1. Cast Iron
2. High—Temperature Stainless Steel
3. High—Temperature Glass—Pyrex
4. Earthenware Ceramic Cookware
5. Glass
6. Bamboo
7. Plastic—only for cold foods and cold storage, including freezers. Not for cooking or reheating.

FAMILY AND FRIENDS

One of my favorite memories growing up was Wednesday night dinner at my grandma's house. Imagine this scene: At least four generations of family members, including great-grandparents, grandparents, moms, dads, uncles, aunts, cousins, brothers, sisters, and a whole lot of brothers from another mother (if you know what I mean). At a typical Wednesday night at my grandma's house, you would find twenty to fifty people laughing and carrying on.

Kids would play outside until we were called inside to set the dinner table and eat. Some of the older kids usually would help out in the kitchen, learning the family secrets for making things taste so good. Every woman would make her signature dish with the understanding that no other woman would even attempt to top it—all out of respect for how delicious the dish was to eat. Some of the men would gather around the TV, paying it no mind and talking over it, of course. There would be smells coming from the kitchen that would make Louisiana proud that her spirit still burned bright.

In the kitchen, there was a little table with a radio playing the latest Stevie Wonder or Marvin Gaye or Michael Jackson. It was a golden time to be alive. On the yellow walls, I remember three bronze Jell-O molds in the shape of fish. I don't remember the molds ever being used.

Now, around the little table where the music played, were three or four seats where different people would sit, trying to steal a taste of what was bubbling, boiling, or frying on the stove. What a scene—like something from a movie—and I lived it. Wow, I miss everything about it. Especially the people, most of whom have long since passed. It was a golden time to be a child. I learned then that a home filled with food, folks, and laughter is a home filled with love. I also learned that love has a flavor and its flavor, is heard in the sound…Ummmmmmmmm.

The food wasn't very alkalizing, believe me. But it did have something else in it that you could only know was there when you closed your eyes after a bite and felt it. It had love energy in every bite, because every bite made me say "Ummmmmmm." Well almost every bite—I wasn't that fond of the lima beans. But as I close my eyes and write this for you, my body still remembers what Wednesday night dinners at my grandma's house felt like. And believe me when I tell you: Lucky is the person who has a tradition like this to remember from the heart.

Growing up with so many family and friends around, I had no idea how lucky I was—this tradition was just normal, and something we did every Wednesday night. Shouldn't it be that way for all children—normal? It was something I always looked forward to. I don't really know what more to say about this, except that I hope you give yourself the opportunity to create a similar tradition in your life—either for the first time or all over again. It is one of my biggest dreams in life to have Wednesday night dinners return again as my own family tradition. I think I'll start cultivating the energy to create this tradition during my next meditation. I hope you will too.

And here's a little secret: All traditions start with the first time.

BEVERAGES

Beverages are important to consider in any discussion about Eating Healthy, because too often they are overused. Optimal digestion requires healthy amounts of stomach acid at a pH between breakdown into smaller absorbable components. A popular saying in Naturopathic Medicine goes applies here: *You aren't what you eat, you're what you can absorb.* When you drink cold beverages in excess of 8 ounces, you essentially dilute your stomach acid and make the digestion process much more difficult. Cold beverages and drinking too much can set the stage for acid reflux and indigestion because of how they inactivate stomach acid.

For this reason, it is best to limit beverages during major meals to small alkalizing drinks of less than 8 ounces during the meal. *Your digestion works best when you consume your largest beverages at least two hours before or after—not during—a major meal.*

Some of the best beverages to drink when Eating Healthy include clean water, herbal teas, espressos, and freshly made vegetable and fruit juices. Remember to keep them at room temperature or warmer, and to drink just enough to clear your palate.

TOTAL CALORIES

It's difficult to put on weight without eating more calories than you burn. Did you know that as of 1985, not one single state in the United States had an obese population higher than 15 percent? As of 2009, there isn't one single state in the United States that has an obese population lower than 20 percent. Thirty-three have an obese population greater than 25 percent. This creates an enormous burden—not only for the physical body, but also for state and federal financial resources. A sick society is an economically broken society.

Below are two very disturbing trends in our country for American adults and our children.

I hope these numbers speak for themselves. Nearly 75 percent of adults in this country are overweight or considered morbidly obese, and nearly 50 percent of our children are obese. America—it's time to take a look in the mirror, a look in the kitchen, and then back in the mirror again.

Clearly, the idea of three square meals is not working. And clearly, the excessive consumption of refined sugar, pesticides, tainted meat, and lack of exercise is not working either. Every $1 out of $10 spent on healthcare in America is spent on treating diabetes. As of 2007, there were more than 18 million diagnosed cases of diabetes, with an estimated 5.7 million cases that are still undiagnosed. Additionally, there are more than 57 million diagnosed cases of pre-diabetes. As of 2007, America spent $174 billion dollars on diagnosed diabetes care alone. Then if you count the undiagnosed cases along with the pre-diabetic diagnoses, the figure skyrockets to $218 billion, according to the American Diabetes Association. All of this continues to trend upward. Since we started recording statistics related to diabetes and obesity, we have not had one year that has shown a decline in either area. And yet, people complain about illegal immigrants and government waste! Perhaps it's time we looked in the mirror. Real change begins with the individual.

Percentage of Adult Population Currently Living at an Unhealthy Weight

National Health and Nutrition Examination Study (NHANES) courtesy of the Centers for Disease Control (CDC)			
Adults older than 20	1960—1962	1988—1994	2007—2008
% of Americans Overweight	31.5	32.2	33.6
% of Americans Obese	13.4	23.2	34.3
% of Americans Morbidly Obese	0.9	3.0	6.0
% of Total Population Overweight, Obese, or Morbidly Obese	45.8%	58.4%	73.9%

Percentage of Children Currently Living at an Unhealthy Weight

National Health and Nutrition Examination Study (NHANES) courtesy of the Centers for Disease Control (CDC)			
Children and Adolescents	1971—1974	1988—1994	2007—2008
% 2—5 years old Obese	5.0	7.2	10.4
% 6—11 years old Obese	4.0	11.3	19.6
% 12—19 years old Obese	6.1	10.5	18.1
% of Total Population Obese	15.1%	29.0%	48.1%

Does the need to clearly define what Eating Healthy is make more sense now? I sure hope that it does. So now we come to the **Principle of Advanced Natural Medicine #18**: *Burn every calorie you consume every day.*

Benefits of Eating Healthy—Energy-Cultivating Emotions

From your body's perspective, the main reason for Eating Healthy is to create Alkaline Cellular Environments and the nutrient density needed for optimal production of energy in your Mitochondria. Of the sixteen factors associated with Eating Healthy, each one of them has a direct link back to the Mitochondria and energy production.

The benefits of Eating Healthy include having more energy and holding less pollution in your body. But how do you really know that these changes are having a positive effect?

Look no further than Energy-Cultivating Emotions (see **Figure 2.2**). In chapter 2, we first revealed the energetic connection that exists between nutrients, tastes, organs, and emotions. It is important to understand that emotion is directly linked to the health of a particular organ. If, for example, your Liver cells are challenged by alcohol, pesticides, and hormones found in conventional industrial meat, then the stage is set for Energy-Draining Reactions such as anger, mood swings, frustration, complaining, and impatience. Conversely, if your Liver cells are supported by Organic carrots, legumes, and turmeric, then there is a strong likelihood that Energy-Cultivating Responses like patience, contentment, and a sense of peace will result.

Eating Healthy promotes Alkaline Cellular Environments and greater energy production. The combination of alkalinity and greater energy production results in a body that feels better, and Energy-Cultivating Responses. In other words, there is a strong correlation between what we eat and how we feel.

Benefits of a Calorie Restriction Lifestyle

Consume. Consume. Consume. When you spend any amount of time thinking about the goals of the incessant advertising we are subjected to, this can be the only conclusion to arrive at. With every commercial we watch, every radio ad we listen to, every print ad we read, the message is always the same—to consume.

With respect to our daily diet, we are taught to consume three large meals each day, which means something drastically different today than it did decades ago. In 1960, the average dinner plate was nine inches in diameter, and the meals had approximately 800 calories. At that time, we were encouraged consume a slightly high, but still relatively healthy 2,400 calories. These numbers were destined to rise as marketing began to encourage more consumption. By the late 1980s, the average dinner plate had grown to 10 inches in diameter, and was able to hold approximately 1,000 calories—meaning we were being asked to consume at least 3,000 calories each day. By 2000, the average dinner plate morphed into an 11-inch model, and had a greater curvature that could hold 1,600 calories. Americans were being asked to consume 4,800 calories each day. But why stop there when more consumption leads to higher profits? By 2010, the average plate size had grown to 12 inches in diameter, with the ability to hold 1,900 calories. That's enough space to hold a minimum of 5,700 calories each day, not counting seconds or thirds. Astounding!

In America, we have been taught to clean our plates. In 1960, eating a plate full of food three times each day meant the consumption of 2,400 calories. A little over fifty years later, cleaning your plate three times a day leads to the consumption of a whopping 5,700 calories a day. It is recommended that an adult needs between 1,800 and 2,400 calories a day to support optimal metabolic functioning. But according to a USDA survey, the average American consumes 4,270 calories each day. In my practice, I have observed that for my adult patients to look and feel perfectly healthy, they need about 2,000 calories or less each day to maintain their weight. So with current eating trends and plate sizes, it's not difficult to see that we are simply consuming WAY too much food. In fact, most of our diseases are directly related to overconsumption—including the overconsumption of refined sugar, pesticides, and polluted conventional industrial meat.

If you consume more calories than you use each day, then the only outcome that can result is weight gain. Here is yet another case where more is NOT better—better is better.

When we look at the benefits of a calorie-restricted lifestyle, it's important to make note of a couple of things. First and foremost, *this is a lifestyle, not a diet.* Secondly, it's important to understand that hunger is your body's way of searching for nutrients and fuel. In fact, when your body is deficient in the nutrients that are essential for energy production, it will tell you that you are hungry. When your nutritional requirements are satisfied, your stomach will be satisfied and hunger will go away. If you are choosing nutrient-deficient foods, then you will need to eat more to satisfy your body's nutritional requirements, which results in the inevitable consumption of excess calories. That's the way it works.

If your food is devoid of nutrients, then your body will need more food. If your food is nutrient dense, then your body will need less of it.

The calorie-restricted lifestyle is very easy to follow, and a wonderful way to reduce calorie consumption into healthy ranges.

STEP 1

Follow the guidelines for Eating Healthy.

STEP 2

Eat one major meal each day before 3 P.M. with family and friends.

STEP 3

Eat one light meal with family and friends.

STEP 4

Eat several healthy alkalizing snacks throughout the day as needed.

STEP 5

Supplement with essential Mitochondrial nutrients four to five times a week.

Following this simple plan will reduce your total daily calorie consumption to a healthy nutrient-dense range below 2,000 calories each day—without having to experience the hunger pains that so often derail good intentions when it comes to losing excess weight. *The scientific support for a calorie-restricted lifestyle is based on studies of Rhesus monkeys that showed that calorie restriction improves life span and quality of life by significantly reducing the incidence and age of the onset of disease.* Essentially, eat less and look forward to living longer—all while enjoying a much happier experience. This is not rocket science.

On a final note, because you will be eating less, you will be able to reallocate your budget to purchase Organic foods, while still saving money each month for investments, savings, and fun family trips. Certainly, pregnant women will need a much higher caloric intake for the simple fact that it takes up to 75,000 calories to grow a baby in the womb. Children will also need two to three large meals each day, but once they're grown, three large meals will make them grow out, not up. The **Principle of Advanced Natural Medicine #19** is this: *An adult body needs only one major meal each day to thrive energetically.*

Example of a Calorie-Restricted Day

Time	Activity	Calories Consumed	Calories Burned
11P.M.—7A.M.	Sleeping and Nice Dreams		496
7A.M.—7:15A.M.	Morning Bowel Movement, Brush Teeth		46
7:15A.M.—8:15A.M.	Alkalizing Breathing Exercises		242
8:15A.M.—9A.M.	Organic A.M. Light Meal: *two pieces of toast, two slices free-range turkey bacon, Organic Eggs, Antioxidant Smoothie, Mitochondrial Nutrients*	682	
9A.M.—12P.M.	Work and Herbal Tea	8	401
12P.M.—1P.M.	Organic Major Meal: *Bowl of Free-Range Chicken Tortilla Soup with Avocados, Grilled Eggplant and Zucchini, Flour Tortilla, Steamed Spinach, Quinoa Cookie, Carrot and Orange Juice*	1,352	
1P.M.—4P.M.	Work and Water		401
4P.M.—4:15P.M.	Organic Snack: *Almonds*	422	
4:15P.M.—6P.M.	Work		214
6P.M.—7P.M.	Exercise or Play		356
7P.M.—8P.M.	Organic Snack: *Small Spinach Salad or Fruit, something easy to digest*	92	
8P.M.—11P.M.	Family Time and Work Preparation for next day		342
TOTALS	**Alkalizing Day**	**2,556**	**2,498**

For the purposes of this example, note that 2,500 calories is still a fairly large amount of calories to consume in one day, with most sedentary people needing only about 1,500 to 2,000 a day to function optimally well. The difference here is due in large part to the suggested activity level.

In this example, notice how the major meal occurs before 3 P.M. to allow for complete digestion of the largest meal well before bedtime. Also notice how the number of calories consumed roughly equals the total number of calories burned. As a good rule to live by, burning what you consume is the most healthy way to go.

Benefits of Organic Juicing, Antioxidant Smoothies, Herbal Teas

I have several simple rules I follow to ensure I'm Eating Healthy without cramping my busy, professional lifestyle. Certainly, I practice calorie restriction and each of the principles we've highlighted in this chapter—especially eating something green every day.

Most mornings, it is common to find me enjoying an ORAC Antioxidant beverage after breathing practice, meditation, and prayer. This is a way for me to start my day right, by giving me and my body everything it needs to be successful—oxygen, peace of mind, remembering what I am about, and all the essentials for Mitochondrial Energy Production. With a start like this, I can accomplish at least two healing goals. First, I fill myself with positive energy so that I have positive energy to give to everyone I interact with throughout the day. Yep, 'me' time comes first every day—an act of benevolent selfishness. Second, I give myself more room for error in case I encounter someone with negative energy, so that I can let it go around me like an unpleasant breeze without taking on any of the negative energy. Becoming frustrated, angry, or anxious is a choice. Giving to yourself first on multiple levels ensures that you have the clarity of mind to make the best choices throughout your day. Build that positive momentum in your life from the moment you wake up.

On a final note, foods with a high concentration of nutrients can be considered medicine. Organic juicing, antioxidant smoothies, and herbal teas are a great way to give your body natural medicine every morning. What's better for your body in the morning—a glass of Organic juice or a doughnut?

Every kitchen should have a juicer for juicing, a blender for making smoothies, a stainless steel or ceramic tea pot, and a French press. My favorite juicer has been the Green Star for the last decade, but a Champion or any juicer also is great to own. For a high-end blender, you might consider owning a VitaMix, which is especially effective for preparing raw and vegan dishes. But again, any blender will do. A French press is a quick way of making and steeping coffee. But here's the thing—coffee is an herb, so you can put any blend of herbs you like in a French press to easily make herbal teas without the hassle of tea balls, tea bags, and all that jazz.

If you are diabetic, pre-diabetic, or working to lose weight, these recipes will likely do more harm than good because of their high sugar content. As such, each should be avoided in favor of your Naturopathic Doctor's recommendations.

When enjoying an Organic juice, antioxidant smoothie, or herbal tea, it is best practice to drink them over the course of thirty minutes to an hour to prevent a potential sugar rush.

ORGANIC ANTIOXIDANT JUICE RECIPES

The A and C Half and Half

- 4—7 Large Organic Carrots
- 4—7 Organic Oranges, Blood Oranges, or Tangerines
- Add a bulb of Ginger in the Winter to spice it up

The I Love My Liver

- 4—7 Large Organic Carrots
- 3—4 Organic Celery Stalks
- ½ Organic Red Beet
- 3—4 Leaves of Organic Kale or Dino Kale
- 1 Bulb of Ginger
- ½—1 Organic Apple (Fujis or Honeycrisps are the best)
- Optional 1—2 ounces of Organic Wheatgrass as a Chaser

ORGANIC ANTIOXIDANT SMOOTHIE RECIPE

The Blueberry Blast

- ½—1 Cup of Frozen Organic Blueberries (*Strawberries, Blackberries, or Mixed Berries are great too!*)
- 1 Cup of Organic Unfiltered Apple Juice (*Pineapple, Mango, and Coconut Juice are great too!*)
- ½ Cup of Organic Oat Milk (*Almond, Soy, Rice, and Hemp Milk are great too!*)
- ½ Organic Banana if desired
- ½—1 cup of spring water to for thinning to desired consistency
- **Blend and Enjoy!**

You also may want to add the following nutrients after blending:

- Chlorella, Spirulina, or other Green Superfoods
- Rice or Pea Protein Powder
- Bee Pollen if not allergic to bee products
- Lecithin Powder
- Extra Quercetin

Dr. Henele's Antioxidant AM Tea®

- Organic Spearmint Leaves—4 parts
- Organic Peppermint Leaves—1.5 parts
- Organic Nettle Leaves—2 parts
- Organic Green Tea—0.75 parts
- Organic Cut Rose Hips—1 part
- Organic Black Elderberries—0.75 parts
- Organic Hawthorn Berries—1.5 parts
- Organic Chaga—1 part
- Organic Cut Licorice Root—3.5 parts
- Organic Burdock Root—2 parts
- Organic Rosemary—1 part
- **1 Tablespoon per cup of distilled water. Steep for 10 minutes in French press before enjoying.**

STAPLES VERSUS INDULGENCES

Is it possible to practice all sixteen aspects of Eating Healthy every meal, every day, and not go a little crazy? The answer to that would probably be no.

Think about meals outside of the house and parties with your friends and family—who wants to miss those special times, or even worse, have to bring your own food to the party. That's a little rude don't you think? There are some occasions throughout the year where the reins are going to have to come off, so to speak, or at least get loosened. That's completely understandable and reasonable.

The practice of Eating Healthy is not meant to be restrictive or frustrating. It is meant to help maximize your body's daily production of energy so that you can feel awesome. Along the way, it will give you a much greater room for error during the infrequent times you wish to indulge. After all, food is meant to be enjoyed and celebrated in the company of the ones we love most. Eating Healthy is a practice that is based on the concept of staples and indulgences.

A **staple** is a food or beverage that can be safely eaten at any meal every day of the month, without any concern about inhibiting your Mitochondrial ability to produce energy. An **indulgence** is a food that breaks one or more of the sixteen Eating Healthy Guidelines and inhibits your Mitochondrial ability to produce energy—often by creating Acidic Cellular Environments. While staples are healthy every day and every meal, indulgences are best limited to no more than two to four days per month, refraining from back-to-back days whenever possible. There are two annual situations where the number of indulgent days per month will probably be greater than two days—during family vacations, and during the holiday season in December.

Everyone I have ever worked with who has committed to Eating Healthy has enjoyed it so much that they seldom stray from the guidelines. And when they do, they get a chance to feel what the foods from their previous lifestyle were really doing to them. People who overconsume calories, sugar, pesticides, hormones, and the like become numb to the damage the foods are actually causing. So it is a good idea to stray occasionally so you can continue to appreciate the great changes you have made by practicing Eating Healthy.

Should Dairy Be a Staple of My Diet?

The simple answer is no, definitely not. This also includes Organic milk. Before we even get into what's in milk, let's examine a couple of facts.

First, dairy includes all of the following—cow milk, cow yogurt, cheese, ice cream, butter, casein, whey, and any product with milk in it.

Second, dairy is in the top four of the most common Delayed Food Allergies, with the other three being gluten, eggs, and yeast.

Third, humans are the only species on the planet that consume milk after 7 years of age.

Fourth, humans are the only species that consume the milk of another species.

Fifth, mother's milk is specifically designed with the correct percentage of protein, fats, colostrum, growth hormone, and immunoglobulins (antibodies) for the energetic needs of a growing baby of the same species.

When you put these five simple facts together, it must raise an eyebrow at least once.

So let's raise the other eyebrow, shall we?

What's In My Moo Juice?

1. **Up to 750,000 Pus Cells per mL** (1/5th of a teaspoon)
2. **rBGH**—Bovine Growth Hormone
3. **Antibiotics**
4. **MTBE**—Rocket Fuel
5. **Pesticides**
6. **GMOs**—Genetically Modified Organisms
7. **Naturally Occurring Hormones** designed specifically for an animal that will grow to be 1,000 to 1,500 pounds.

Pus Cells. Pus. Pus. Pus Cells. Yummy.

Did you know I'm purposely working to gross you out? Good. Did you know that any milk with more than 200 million pus cells per liter is not recommended for human consumption? Did you know that of the 50 states in the Union, only Hawaii currently produces milk with less than 200 million pus cells per liter?

Did you know that a pus cell is a concentration of immune cells from the cow, glycoaminoglycan complexes similar to acne, bacterial infections, blood, and antibiotic resistant germs? *Yes. When you pour a bowl of milk you are essentially pouring acne all over your highly refined sugar morning breakfast cereal. When you grab that morning cup of coffee, you are adding liquid acne to your get-up-and go.* How can anyone expect to be healthy eating another animal's pus?

So here's the secret. When you add enough sugar to anything it tastes GREAT! As a doctor, how can I recommend to anyone that a food with all of these drawbacks is a healthy staple of their diet? Can you safely eat it as a very infrequent indulgence? Sure. Who doesn't like pizza? For as crappy as that indulgence is, it tastes really, really good. But should the poison that is dairy be going into your body several times a day, every day of your life? Absolutely, if you fancy drinking another animal's pus.

Anyway, do that when we live in a day and age where there are so many wonderful alternatives?

You like cereal? Great! Use an alternative milk as your staple. Most people love Organic oat milk, but there's also Organic rice, soy, almond, hemp, coconut, hazelnut, and other milks for your cereal and coffee.

You like to bake or a recipe calls for milk? Great! Use an alternative milk. It works in a one-to-one ratio, and is a fantastic replacement for cow milk.

You like cheese? Great! Try a casein-free nut cheese or raw cheese as a staple of your diet. Or simply eat it on your indulgent days during the month.

You like yogurt or ice cream? Great! Try coconut-, soy-, or rice-based products. I love ice cream, and I hated giving it up to tell you the truth—until I tasted chocolate coconut ice cream. Now I could care less about cow ice cream.

You like butter? Great! Use coconut oil or an Organic oil-based spread that you can find in any local store. Tastes just the same, and it's healthy for you too.

You like whey protein powders? Great! Switch to a rice- or pea-based protein powder. I can't tell you how many people I've seen who are on a whey protein powder until I test them for Delayed Food Allergies and we find out that their sinus congestion and aches and pains were because of the whey. Just because someone tells you something is good for you, doesn't mean that it's good for you.

My point is that there are a ton of delicious alternatives, with more choices available every day to help us break some of our awful habits.

There are a million ways to avoid pus in your breakfast.

At no time on Earth have humans consumed five servings of dairy each day, and lived to tell a healthy tale. So I guess because of all our fancy technology today, we're somehow exempt? Please.

Should I Drink Tap or Bottled Water?

Anyone worried about what I might say for this topic? Or are you still recovering from the acne corn flakes? God, I love this stuff! Take heart—as I've always promised, I will never slam something without providing an easy and healthy alternative that also saves you money.

First, a short list of what's in tap water that you will most definitely want to avoid.

What's In My Tap Water?

1. **Fluoride**—Binds Magnesium essential for ATP Production.
2. **Lead**—Binds to bone tissue, and inhibits the formation of healthy Red Blood Cells that are essential for carrying oxygen and managing blood pH.
3. **Aluminum**—Destroys the Electron Transport Chain in Mitochondria.
4. **Chlorine and Chloroform**
5. **Bacteria, Viruses, and other Microorganisms**
6. **MTBE**—Rocket Fuel
7. **Pesticides**
8. **Antibiotics, Antidepressants, and Medications** for Blood Pressure, High Cholesterol, Pain, and other conditions.

Most municipal tap water is a combination of water from streams, rivers, lakes, and underground aquifers. Did you know that as of 2008 it is projected that more than 250 million pounds of medical grade waste is produced each year, including pharmaceuticals? It also is estimated that more than a quarter of this waste is dumped by health-service facilities and patients at home each year. So one might ask, how do antibiotics, antidepressants, and other pharmaceuticals get into tap water?

The answer is in reclaimed and treated water. After your toilet flushes or water goes down a drain, most municipalities will reclaim the water and treat it in an attempt to purify it. Reclaimed and treated water is supposed to be used exclusively for landscaping and agricultural endeavors because it is classified as non-potable. However, that is not always the case. Reclaimed and treated water also can be used to replenish the very underground aquifers that supply a portion of your tap water.

What this means is that when you drink or cook with tap water, you are potentially drinking a treated remnant of anything that goes into a toilet. The Environmental Working Group has compiled a database of tap water from every major municipality in the country. As of 2004, their research has uncovered more than 300 pollutants in American tap water. Will a water filter make this better? A little, but isn't it like trying to make a silk purse out of a sow's ear?

So, what can you do about it?

The National Resources Defense Council (www.NRDC.org) compiled a wonderful study of bottled waters, and it is the best one produced to date. For the study, the council randomly purchased bottled waters and had them independently tested for plastic residue, bacteria, and heavy metals. What they uncovered were the following high-quality, safe bottled waters.

Ranking of Safe Bottled Waters

1. Ice Age®
2. Hawaiian Springs®, FIFI®, Naya®
3. Arrowhead®
4. Smartwater®
5. Evian®
6. San Pellegrino®
7. Crystal Geysers®
8. DASANI®, Aquafina®

While many new bottled waters have come to market over the last several years, there is not a lot of data from independent lab testing. When discussing bottled waters, there also is the concern about many bottled waters being nothing more than tap water, and the growing concern about plastics ending up in landfills. I only recommend the bottled waters on the list above, and please make sure to recycle your empty bottles. Your body is two-thirds to three-quarters water, so water is an essential aspect of Eating Healthy and worth the $30 to $60 each month it takes to replenish your body with clean H20.

Your body will need approximately half of your body weight in fluid ounces of water every day. So, for example, if you weigh 100 pounds, you will need 50 fluid ounces of clean water every day, and slightly more on days that you sweat.

Finally, it is a good idea to transport your water in a glass jar or stainless steel container that is free of Bisphenol A (BPA). If you're like me, you have a tendency to leave your bottle of water in your vehicle during the day. Water in a Polyethylene terephthalate (PETE) 1, PETE 2, or PETE 7 plastic container that is subjected to 80-degree temperatures or direct sunlight can begin to transfer plastics (phthalates) into the water, and breakdown the Electro Transport Chain of your Mitochondria.

Is My Microwave Safe?

Microwaves are technically safe, but not recommended as a usual method of cooking or reheating because of the effect it has on amino acid peptide bonds. Amino acids are linked by peptide bonds to form proteins in what closely resembles a string of pearls. Each pearl would be an amino acid and the string would be the peptide bonds. Microwaving causes peptide bonds to shrink much more than cooking at low to medium temperatures on a stove, grill, or even in the oven. The results are amino acids that are very close together, and as a result, difficult to breakdown in your stomach. Microwaving makes your digestive system work much harder to digest a meal.

Additionally, many microwave-safe dishes are plastic. Heating plastics leaches harmful phthalates into the food or beverage. Phthalates disrupt female and male reproductive Physiology. Anyone in the mood for some Endometriosis or a little Erectile Dysfunction?

Where to Shop

When I think of grocery shopping, I think of Whole Foods, Sprouts, and local Farmer's Markets. It is easy to find a cornucopia (can't write a chapter about nutrition without using that word at least once) of great Organic foods, produce, and free-range meats at these locals. In fact, it can be quite a fun experience for the whole family. I encourage you to take your children with you as you shop, and that you allow them to help prepare your meals. Include the kids — teach them how to shop, cook, clean. Involve them from the time they're able to burp so they develop lifelong skills for self-care. Kids love to learn, and you can enjoy a break once they are old enough. Imagine nights where the kids make the meals. It can happen when you invest in them early on.

For a great list of local Farmers Markets in your area, check out NRDC.org at http://www.simplesteps.org/eat-local/farmers-markets.

Farmers Markets are a great secret for taking the entire family out on a weekend morning. I've been going for years, and I haven't had a bad experience yet.

Documentaries and Text Resources

Below are a few resources that I strongly recommend. Most of the DVDs can be viewed for free on YouTube, Hulu, or on demand through Netflix.

Documentaries

- *Food Inc.*—Simply a must-see documentary! Watch it on a Tuesday night because it can be a bit of a downer. But it is an essential movie to see that can help you make the right decisions regarding your diet. Why Tuesday? Because at least the next day is hump day.
- *The Botany of Desire*
- *Super Size Me*
- *Our Daily Poison*
- *The World According to Monsanto*
- *The Future of Food*

Texts

- *The World's Healthiest Foods*—George Mateljan
- *Healing With Whole Foods*—Paul Pitchford

Listening to Your Amazing Body

So much to do and so little time to do it in. Or maybe it just seems that way. Remember to take changes one step at a time. Have fun with all of this. You can decide to make it too overwhelming and raise the white flag, or you can decide to have fun with it and try something new for a couple of weeks before moving onto the next thing you want to incorporate into your life. New lifestyles are evolved into. Take your time, and enjoy the ride.

EATING HEALTHY GUIDELINES

The following questionnaire is designed to help you get a feel for where you can focus your attention with Eating Healthy. The best places to start are where you feel unsure—one aspect at a time. In fact, it might be worthwhile to use this questionnaire as a way to track what you eat for one week, and then answer the following questions. Each time you eat something, check off a number so by the end of the week you can see where you are at with Eating Healthy.

1. How many times per week do you take in all the nutrients essential for Mitochondrial Energy Production?

   0 1 2 3 4 5 6 7 7+ Unsure

2. How many times per week do you eat Organic Sourced Foods?

   0 1 2 3 4 5 6 7 7+ Unsure

3. How many times per week do you eat known Delayed Food Allergens?

   0 1 2 3 4 5 6 7 7+ Unsure

4. How many of your meals are 60 percent Alkalizing each week?

   0 1 2 3 4 5 6 7 7+ Unsure

5. How many times do you eat a Green Food each week?

   0 1 2 3 4 5 6 7 7+ Unsure

6. How many Organic Fruits, Vegetables, Beans, Juices, Smoothies, or Herbal Teas do you eat/drink each week?

   0 1 2 3 4 5 6 7 7+ Unsure

7. How many of your meals have less than 8 grams of Refined Sugar each week?

   0 1 2 3 4 5 6 7 7+ Unsure

8. How many times each week do you satisfy your sweet craving with an Organic fruit?

   0 1 2 3 4 5 6 7 7+ Unsure

9. How many of your meals have more than 8 grams of Fiber each week?

   0 1 2 3 4 5 6 7 7+ Unsure

10. How many times do you eat raw fruit, vegetables, or nuts each week?

    0 1 2 3 4 5 6 7 7+ Unsure

11. How many meals are prepared using Healthy Preparation Methods each week?

    0 1 2 3 4 5 6 7 7+ Unsure

12. How many meals include either Free-Range Meat or Alaskan Wild-Caught seafood each week?

    0 1 2 3 4 5 6 7 7+ Unsure

13. How many meals do you prepare using Environmentally Safe Cookware each week?

    0 1 2 3 4 5 6 7 7+ Unsure

14. How many meals are prepared with the help of Family and/or Friends each week?

    0 1 2 3 4 5 6 7 7+ Unsure

15. How many meals feature a small alkalizing Beverage, 8 ounces or less each week?

    0 1 2 3 4 5 6 7 7+ Unsure

16. How many times were you able to burn off all the Total Calories from a meal on the same day?

    0 1 2 3 4 5 6 7 7+ Unsure

ADDITIONAL QUESTIONS

1. How many times did you eat Fast-food or eat out this week?

   0 1 2 3 4 5 6 7 7+ Unsure

2. How many sodas, energy drinks, or beverages with high-fructose corn syrup or refined sugar did you consume this week? (Count one for every 12 ounces)

   0 1 2 3 4 5 6 7 7+ Unsure

3. How many dairy pus cell products (anything with dairy in it) did you consume this week?

   0 1 2 3 4 5 6 7 7+ Unsure

4. How many times did you eat more than one major meal per day this week?

   0 1 2 3 4 5 6 7 7+ Unsure

5. How many times did you drink or cook with tap water this week?

   0 1 2 3 4 5 6 7 7+ Unsure

6. How many times did you use a microwave this week?

   0 1 2 3 4 5 6 7 7+ Unsure

HOW TO TEST YOUR pH

To perform this test you will need pH test strips. Using a pH test strip record the following test results:

- **Waking A.M. Saliva**
- **First Morning Urine**—Measures the pH of the body's nightly metabolic activity, and any meals consumed within three to four hours of going to bed. Thus, for the most accurate measurement, try to refrain from eating a major meal three to four hours before going to bed.
- **Last Evening Urine**—Measures the pH changes in the body throughout the day. This measurement is tied to the foods and beverages you have consumed throughout the day, as well as the amount of stress you had experienced during the day.

Notes:

1. If using pH test strips, remember that the results must be read within fifteen to thirty seconds.
2. To accurately test for saliva pH, be sure to record the finding before eating, drinking, or brushing your teeth.

Interpretation:

- Saliva below 5.5 = Very Acidic. Replenish Minerals, and Use Alkalizing Water Sources.
- Saliva between 5.6–6.0 = Slightly Acidic. Replenish Minerals, and Use Alkalizing Water Sources.
- **Saliva between 6.1–6.9 = Optimal pH Range.**
- Saliva greater than 7.0 = Too Alkaline. Possible Testing Error.
- Urine below 6.0 = Very Acidic. Replenish Minerals, and Use Alkalizing Water Sources.
- **Urine between 6.1 and 6.9 = Optimal pH ranges. Vitamin and mineral reserves are healthy.**
- Urine greater than 7.0 = Possible Reactive Alkalosis from severe mineral depletion, or a diet that is too Alkaline.

To determine if your diet is alkaline or acidic, we would compare the First Morning Urine reading with the Last Evening Urine reading. If the pH increases, then your diet is alkaline, but if the pH lowers, then your diet is probably acidic. For example consider the following readings: First Morning Urine 6.4; Last Evening Urine 6.8. These reading would suggest that the foods you ate throughout the day were alkaline for your body.

To determine if your body has the most optimal pH for healing, we would compare the prior Last Evening's Urine with the next First Morning Urine reading. The pH should stay relatively stable, and should be within the 6.1 to 7.0 range. For example consider the following reading: Tuesday Last Evening Urine 6.2; Wednesday First Morning Urine 6.4. These readings indicate that your body is in the optimal pH range for healing during the night while you sleep.

What You Can Do To Cultivate Energy Today

There's literally so much to do with Eating Healthy and all of the various aspects that it should be easy to select a change or two and begin making improvements. That said, let me present several options that most people find very fun to explore. Feel free to explore them all—you will not be disappointed.

1. **Try a New Market**—Do the family shopping in a new store like a Whole Foods, Sprouts, or other health food store. (I laugh when I hear things like health food store or health food aisle—or even health food—because shouldn't all stores, aisles, and food be healthy?)

2. **Take the Organic Challenge**—Make two meals on the same night for the family. Make one meal with 100 percent Organic ingredients, and the other all conventional ingredients—complete with pesticides and antibiotics. Let the family enjoy a blind taste test to discover which meal rocks.

3. **Try a New Milk**—You deserve a pus-free milk. Select one or more of the following milks to sample: Oat, Almond, Soy, Rice, Coconut, Hemp, Hazelnut, or Multigrain. Chill Them, Drink Them. Cook with Them. Find One You Like.

4. **Try a Local Farmers Market**—Use the resource provided earlier in this chapter to find a nearby Farmers Market, take the family, some cash, and go have a blast. Farmers markets are great places to get the best produce, and save a lot of money too.

5. **Eat Something Green Every Day**—Simple as that. This experience is best done over the course of two to three weeks. Let's see how you feel after that.

6. **Lose Some Calories**—Practice a Calorie-Restriction Lifestyle. One Major Meal each day, One Light Meal, and a couple of alkalizing snacks, water, Organic juice, smoothie, or herbal tea. That's it. No refined sugars, no sodas, no energy drinks, no fast-food, or eating out. Try it for one to three weeks, and let's see how you feel.

ALKALIZING HEALING PLAN

	Therapy	**Instructions**
Primary Therapy	Organic Clinical Nutrition	Explore your Eating Healthy improvement.
Complementary Therapy	Breathing Practice	Upon waking and before starting your morning routine, breathe for fifteen to thirty minutes. Listen to your breath on the inhale and exhale. Get stronger.
Complementary Therapy	Yoga	Activate your feet frequently throughout the day while standing, walking, or sitting.
Complementary Therapy	Exercise	Exercise using whatever method or variety of methods you choose. The goal is a minimum of thirty minutes from the time you begin to perspire, three to five times this week.
Essential Therapy	Sunlight	Take breaks frequently throughout your workday to go outside and enjoy some sunshine on your face.
Essential Therapy	Positive Internal Dialogue	Finding Something Good. Before you go to sleep, reflect on four things that happened during your day that made you feel good. During your day when you find yourself thinking about something stressful, Change It. Find What's Good.

7. **Choose Any of the Eating Healthy Guidelines**—Put them into practice for at least a week to get a feel for them. But to really feel their benefits, explore them for two to four weeks. Keep the ones that work for you. The ones that don't keep those too—until they work for you.

RESOLUTION #7

Watch *Food, Inc.*

RESOLUTION #8

Select any of the fun Eating Healthy improvements and try them out. Information without action is only wishing on a star—and that won't get the Mitochondria crankin.'

Eating Healthy improvement I will explore this week:

____

Acidic Food or Beverage I will give up this week:

____

HEALING JOURNAL RECORDING

Record in your Healing Journal your moods, thoughts, and positive experiences throughout the week. Pay special attention to how you are dealing with the changes in your diet, and what you are feeling about some of the things you have read in this chapter. Keep developing your ability to spend more time thinking about What's Good.

Good Luck!

CHAPTER 6: THE ART OF ENERGETICS

Learning Your Body in a New Way

Interesting Insights to look for in this chapter:

- The *Change It* recipe.
- Emotions that cultivate energy… emotions that drain energy.
- How feeling overwhelmed starts with overwhelming your digestion.
- What red eyes reveal about your Liver.

Principle of Advanced Natural Medicine #20:
Health is our ability to maximize the unification of our genetic potential with the energetic potential of our spirit, so as to achieve the personal development necessary to realize our dreams in this lifetime.

What If?

What if your body was pre-wired to integrate every single cell with every other cell in an incredible, multi-dimensional pathway for communication? What if these pathways allowed for the health of an organ to influence the health of a Joint, or a Tendon, or a Muscle? What if these pathways responded to changes in emotion, to the food you ate, to how your body moved and even various postures. What if you realized that you are far more beautiful and wonderful than you have previously imagined? Would you be interested to learn how your body attempts to communicate with you?

There are no accidents in your body, and much of this is due to the Sophisticated Simplicity we discussed in the previous chapter. But it is also due to the fact that we are Energetic beings.

Energetics is an essential part of the Cycle of Influencing Energy® and a fantastic thought process for understanding how your body is integrated. Your body is made up of cells that form tissues, tissues that form organs, organs that form organ systems, and organ systems that form your body. All of this is tied together, integrated, and monitored by your Nervous System, and the energy pathways that go along with it. Energetics is the study of these pathways, and the associations that are created between the organ and associated parts of the body. Energetics helps relate a variety of emotions, tastes, and seemingly unrelated body parts to specific organs, their Anatomical Structure, Physiological Function, and Biochemical Energy Production. Of these potential relationships—perhaps the most fruitful and easiest to learn—is the connection between organ function, energy production, and emotion.

In fact, because your body performs with Sophisticated Simplicity, there is no difference between emotion and organ function—they are one and the same. In my practice, my goal is to translate a patient's symptoms to determine which organs are being affected. The reason I think in this way is because it engenders the highest rate of success I've ever witnessed. If I know which organs are affected, then I know which nutrients and herbs are indicated for treatment. I know which Organic foods will work as medicine. I know which Complementary Therapies will likely be effective for the Healing Process.

The thought process for Energetics is quite simple really:

1. Listen to what the patient is saying, interpret pertinent lab tests and physical exams, and then relate the information to specific organs in the patient's body.
2. Select the nutrients, herbs, and Organic foods necessary for Mitochondrial Energy Production and optimal cellular function.
3. Select the appropriate Complementary Therapies, Essential Therapies, and Fine-Tuning Therapies to finalize the healing plan design.
4. Get out of the way.

For example, when I am listening to someone in a healing capacity, it doesn't matter what they are coming in for as long as I can relate it to organs in their body. It doesn't matter whether they are coming in with high cholesterol, adrenal fatigue, or hypothyroid issues. It doesn't matter whether the discussion involves cancer, depression, obesity, anxiety, or frustration with a relationship. I am always listening for the key words that will unlock the relationship and reveal the correct organ. The rationale pertains to assessments of the obstacles and natural treatments, and it helps me figure out what's wrong so that I can select the correct nutrients, herbs, and Organic foods to help make it right. In an effort to make natural healing easier, you need a thought process, and an understanding of how your body is designed to work. Energetics affords you this thought process and it is one that I am thankful to say I have used successfully for many years.

So what if emotion was one of many ways that your body communicates with you? When you utilize Energetics as a thought process, you are expanding your ability to understand how your body is designed to work as a unified whole. One key ingredient is to understand that there is no difference between an emotion and an organ, and that they are really the same thing as far as your body is concerned. The goal of natural therapeutics is to restore balance and, optimal functioning within each organ of the body. So it is of paramount importance to know which organs to target for therapeutic intervention. This idea brings us to **Principle of Advanced Natural Medicine #21**: *When you do something positive for an organ the improved biochemical cellular functioning of that organ will often result in energy-cultivating emotional responses.* Reciprocally, when you practice energy-cultivating positive emotional responses, then the biochemical cellular functioning of the organ associated with the emotional response will benefit. What we think, feel, and say has a profound effect on our health.

Emotion is an essential component of energy production, and perhaps why belief plays such a profound role in healing. A positive outlook is every bit as effective as a nutrient, herb, or natural healing modality. In fact, we have learned that a positive perspective, that belief that you can heal, and encouragement are much more than afterthoughts to the Healing Process. Thinking positively, feeling positive, and speaking positively are considered medicine when one understands the thought process of Energetics.

So when assessing what's going on inside you, refer to the chart provided in **Figure 6.1** to help you interpret what your body is saying to you. Connect what's going on in an organ, and you will unlock the key to utilizing natural therapeutics in a profound way. As you progress through Volume 2 of this series, you will learn many methods from a variety of perspectives to help heal the cells of each individual organ. You will be directly applying the Cycle of Influencing Energy®, the 4 Considerations for Healing, rules for Mitochondrial Energy Production, Eating Healthy, and especially Energetics. Understand that what you do for (or to) one organ, you do for (or to) your body and your life as a whole.

Energy-Cultivating Responses vs. Energy-Draining Reactions

What effect is how I am feeling emotionally having on my body? This is the question that Energetics seeks to answer. Let's go a little deeper into Energetics with the help of Energy-Cultivating Emotions versus Energy Draining Emotions, and look at some pertinent examples for relating an event in the body to an organ. For the remainder of this chapter, you will want to refer repeatedly to **Figure 6.1**.

Energy-Cultivating Emotions, simply stated, are emotions that help the Mitochondria within your cells produce energy. When entering into a Healing Process, an initial healing decision is made that often is based on courage, belief, and a desire to take action for positive change. As the Healing Process ensues, certain skills are necessary to ensure a disciplined adherence to the healing plan. These skills include being encouraging to yourself and to others, developing a Positive Internal Dialogue with yourself, becoming acutely accountable for your actions, and developing an appreciation for life, nature, other people, and yourself. As the healing decision and healing skills become more a part of your life, they open the door for you to utilize the primary healing responses consistently. So, for example, if you are healing from a Liver issue, it would be helpful to mindfully practice patience. It is important to note that each of the primary healing skills have a positive effect on the specific organs and Energetic associations they are linked with.

Energy-Draining Reactions, simply stated, are reactions that we reflexively and habitually go to when we are fatigued. Tragically unaware of what is being done to the body, many people who are already fatigued react poorly to everyday situations. Habitual reactions result in inhibiting energy production within the Mitochondria of the cell by decoupling the Electron Transport Chain. As it pertains to emotion, there often is a degenerative mental process that people go through which, of course, affects how the body performs. The root cause of these degenerative mental processes is Love Pain. Essentially, we are hurt and our rational mind allows us to learn from the situation so that we can attempt to avoid the cause of the hurt in the future. If what we learn affords us the ability to develop Energy-Cultivating Responses, then it was a good lesson. However, if what we learn only teaches us to engage in Energy-Draining Reactions, then this is where problems typically occur in our lives and within the body.

Once hurt, you may have found yourself using a secondary reaction as a means of coping with the situation. Coping is quite healthy, and a natural, safe place to go immediately following the experience of Love Pain—as long as you don't decide to live there and make the reaction a habit. Secondary reactions affect organs that they are associated with, but do not cause significant damage unless they are used as a habitual way of living. So now let's say you choose to delay beginning a Healing Process, what might happen? Secondary reactions can degenerate into third-level reactions. Third-level reactions are behavioral adaptations we make, and they ultimately are signs that a short-lived coping mechanism is becoming an unhealthy habit. Third-level reactions will take their toll on the body over time, and where the toll is taken is no accident—they can be directly attributed to the organ and tissues associated with the reaction.

So now let's say that your behavioral adaptations have resulted in some rather poor decision-making, and that your decisions have led to more painful experiences—some even self-inflicted. At this point, many people become lost in their own thoughts. They have been trying to figure out why things are happening to them, and how to survive in the face of chaos, uncertainty, and the assault of routine human interactions. People who have a difficult time navigating the emotional landscape of life often will mentally degenerate further into habits of blaming others for their troubles, needing to control every aspect of life (hypercontrolling), and/or playing the role of a victim. It is at this point that the person has entered into the fourth-level reactions and has reached a point where they are becoming destructive to themselves as their thought processes begin to destroy their Mitochondria and their ability to produce energy. The major problems with entering this level are the following: Not only does the reaction negatively affect the entire body, but it also becomes a VERY ingrained habit that can be very difficult to unlearn.

At this point, decisions often get even worse, and people who are prone to blame, hypercontrolling behavior, and/or victimization, often begin to isolate themselves from their support networks, as well as life in general. Isolated and without explanation, many people begin to lose faith in life, what they believed they were entitled to, and ultimately in themselves. It is at this dangerous point in the mental degeneration process that the road to a better reality virtually disappears from sight, and a person finds himself or herself alone and unloved. It is at this point that people often enter fifth-level of reactions and become destructive to themselves and to others. Hallmark signs of a person who is shackled to the slavery of reactions include: persistent negative internal dialogue, vindictiveness, irrational behavior, and the tendency to be judgemental.

It is important to note that fourth- and fifth-level reactions are chronic habitual behaviors that significantly damage the entire body. As such, they create enormous stress for the body, but there also can be growth opportunities. It is also important to note that once a person enters into third-, fourth-, and fifth-level reactions, they can easily move around between all three destructive levels. So, understand that emotion is literally energy in motion, and as such, a person can habitually choose to use any of the Energy-Draining Reactions to promote destruction of the self, and as a result, create the opportunity for true healing.

The wonderful opportunity for true healing? Are you serious? Absolutely.

So what's the solution?

Change It.

Figure 6.1

Genesis Energetics - 5 Element Perspective

	Fire	Earth	Gold	Water	Wood	Accessory Fire
Yin Organs	Heart	Spleen-Pancreas	Lungs	Kidneys	Liver	Pericardium[1]
Yang Organs	Small Intestine	Stomach	Large Intestine	Urinary Bladder	Gall Bladder	Triple Heater-HPAxis[2]
Gland	Thymus	Pancreas	Thyroid, Parathyroid	Adrenals, Reproductive	Liver, Reproductive	HPAxis
Energy Draining Reactions			**Acidity - Sympathetic 'Fight or Flight' Dominance**			
Primary Root Cause	Love Pain					
Secondary Reactions (Coping Mechanism)	Unworthy of Joy, Love or Happiness	Excessive Concentration, Being Busy as an Escape	Grief (Extended Sadness)	Lack of Trust	Anger, Indecisiveness, Emotional Instability	Alone, Isolated, Neglected
3rd Level Reactions (Behavior Adaptation)	Resistant to Change, Acceptance of Defeat	Mental Chatter, Easily Overwhelmed	Keeping It Locked Inside, Unable to 'Let Go'	Fear of Unknown, Worry, Anxiety	Frustration, Impatience, Complaining, Timidness	Guilt, Excessive Thought
4th Level Reactions (Destructive to Self)	Blaming Others, Hypercontrolling &/or Victimized Persona					
5th Level Reactions (Destructive to Self & Others)	Negative Internal Dialogue, Irrational, Vindictive &/or Judgmental Persona					
Energy Cultivating Responses			**Alkalinity - Parasympathetic 'Rest & Digest' Balance**			
Healing Decision	Courage, Belief, Taking Action for Positive Change					
Primary Healing Skills	Encouraging, Positive Internal Dialogue, Accountability, Appreciation					
Primary Healing Responses	Loving, Satisfied, Joyful, Enthusiastic, Authentic	Rational Decision Making, Clear & Calm Mind	Forgiving, Truthful, Encouraging, Postive Communication	Trusting in Life's Perfection, Faithful, Belief	Patient, Peaceful, Confident	Investing In Family, Friends, & Passions Creating Community
Primary Nutrients	Mitochondrial Energy Producing Nutrients, Chlorophyll & Organic Foods					
Supportive Nutrients	Vitamin B12, Folic Acid, Vitamin E, Co-Q-10, Magnesium, Taurine, L-Carnitine, Essential Fatty Acids, Amino Acids	Vitamin C, Vitamin K, Calcium, Essential Fatty Acids, Digestive Enzymes, Amino Acids	Vitamin A, Vitamin D, Vitamin E, Vitamin K, Zinc, Probiotics, N-acetyl Cysteine, L-Glutamine , Glutathione	Clean Water, Vitamin C, Vitamin D, Vitamin K, Biotin, Calcium, Magnesium, Potassium, Sodium	Vitamin A, Vitamin C, Vitamin K, Alpha-Lipoic Acid, Taurine, Lecithin, Essential Fatty Acids, Glutathione, Amino Acids	Minerals, Amino Acids, Vitamin D
Botanical Medicines	Hawthorn Berry, Rosemary, Ginkgo Biloba	Peppermint, Spearmint, Ginger, Gentian, Rose Hips	Cordyceps, Licorice Root, Maitake, Astragalus Root, Lauracidin	Siberian Ginseng, Ashwagandha, Schisandra Berry, Nettles	Green Tea, Milk Thistle, Burdock Root, Turmeric, Reishi	Skull Cap, Passion Flower, Kava Kava, Gotu Kola
Associated Facial Features	Tongue	Lips	Nose	Ears	Eyes (Sclera)	Eyes (Iris)
Additional Associations	Voice	Smooth Muscle	Immune System	Reproductive Organs*	Uterus	Body Temperature
Associated Fluids	Sweat	Saliva	Lymph	Urine & Semen	Tears	Cerebral Spinal Fluid
Tissues	Blood Vessels	Skeletal Muscle	Skin, Sinuses, Lymphatics	Bones	Fascia & Sinews**	Dura Mater - Endocrine
Most Active Seasons	Summer	Late Summer	Autumn	Winter	Spring	Early Summer
Most Active Times	H 11a-1p, SI 1p-3p	Sp-P 9a-11a, St 7a-9a	L 3a-5a, LI 5a-7a	K 5p-7p, UB 3p-5p	L 1a-3a, GB 11p-1a	P 7p-9p, TH 9p-11p
Imbalance Climates	Heat	Dampness	Dryness	Cold	Wind	
Energy Directions	South	Center	West	North	East	
Energy Colors	Red	Yellow	White or Blue	Black	Green	
Energy Tastes	Bitter	Sweet	Hot & Spicy	Salty	Sour	

Note A: Nerve Tissue, Brain and Spinal Cord are indicated by each of the 5 elements and additionally in the Conception (Ren) and Governing (Du) Vessels. These tissues most closely mimic the direction and flow of energy through meridians, uniting the whole body.

Note B: Blood is also indicated by each of the 5 elements. 'Where Qi Flows, Blood Goes,' is a foundational philosophy of TCM. Looking at the body's Anatomy, nerve fibers run so are they accompanied by blood vessels. This fact underscores the direct relationship between qi and blood.

1: The Pericardium is most closely associated with Dural Tissue. Dural Tissue, like the Pericardial Sac, have similar protective functions providing a fluid-filled enclosure for important organs. Where as Dural Tissue protects the Brain and Spinal Cord, the Pericardium protects the Heart.

2: The Triple Heater is also referred to as the San Jiao and Triple Warmer. With respect to the Triple Heater's function in Traditional Chinese Medicine, it most closely resembles the Hypothalamus and Pituitary Glands of Western Physiology. As such, the Triple Heater has a governing effect on the endocrine system.

* The Health of the Kidneys are also indicated by the thickness and luster of Head Hair.

** Fascia is the Connective Tissue that envelopes and penetrates each muscle, forming a continuous web commonly referred to as the Myofascial Network. Sinews are Tendons and Ligaments.

Change It and the Mental High Five

Let's create an awesome healing habit together. When you find yourself experiencing an Energy-Draining Reaction apply the following steps to Change It.

Step 1
Breathe Until You Know Exactly How You Want To Respond.

Step 2
Respond Without Need Of Validation.

Step 3
Practice Positive Internal Dialogue—Encourage Yourself.

Step 4
Give Yourself A Mental High Five.

In Step 1, you are using your awareness to exercise perhaps the only freedom you possess—the freedom of perspective. Breathing allows you to slow yourself down and choose how you want to respond. What's the rush to react? If you don't know how you want to respond to a situation, then clearly you are not ready to respond. That's okay. Move onto Steps 3 and 4, and respond later when you are ready. Then do Steps 3 and 4 again.

In Step 2, you are actually responding, and because you have decided *exactly* how you want to respond, this carries its own sense of satisfaction. The only outcome that matters is the one you've created within yourself to cultivate energy. Which bring us to the **Principle of Advanced Natural Medicine #22**: *Anything that leads to satisfaction cultivates healing energy.* So if the response works out, then great—that's the bonus. By responding instead of reacting, you have already won by generating your own satisfaction—free from the need for validation from anyone else.

In Step 3, it is now important to create great new habits, and perhaps none is more important than how you speak to yourself. If you've just done something awesome, give yourself some immediate positive feedback. Tell yourself: Good Job! Fantastic Work! or something similar. *The key is to give yourself positive feedback immediately and to include your name in the praise. Smiles don't hurt either.*

In Step 4, here's how we lock in the positive change so that it becomes easier and easier to do and is also fun. Give yourself a Mental High Five. Heck, give yourself a real High Five too. Now you've slowed yourself down to find an Energy-Cultivating Response, acted on it, and encouraged yourself. You've also reinforced the positive behavioral change with something as simple as a High Five. Celebrate every positive step you make—it builds positive energy and momentum in life.

Remember—what other people think about you is less important than how you feel about yourself. In the story of your life, you always have the leading role. Things aren't going your way? Change It.

Great Job! Here's a High Five from me to you.

Energetics: Fire Element

Yin Organ	Heart
Yang Organ	Small Intestine
Gland	Thymus—Think Immune Cells
Energetic Associations	Voice reveals strength or weakness
Fluids	Sweat clears stagnant Heart energy
Tissues	Blood Vessels
Time	Heart 11 A.M.–1 P.M., Small Intestine 1 P.M.–3 P.M.
Flavor	Bitter
Energy-Draining Reactions	Love Pain, Unworthiness, Resistance, Feeling of Defeat
Energy-Cultivating Responses	Courage, Joyful, Satisfied, Enthusiastic, Loving

What's Interesting?

I have always found it interesting that sweat is associated with the Fire Element, and specifically with the Heart. It's also interesting that studies out of Japan confirm that sweating—using Infrared Sauna Therapy—is associated with drastic improvements in Congestive Heart Failure patients, and also in the overall performance of the Heart muscle.

Life Lessons for Energy Cultivation

Understand that emotions can indicate what is going on internally in the organs, and they also can heal or create disharmony in the organs. Have you ever been in love with someone? Do you remember how your body felt as you were just starting to feel love? Do you remember having that feeling in your belly that was warm and vulnerable? What you were feeling was the Energetic link between your Heart and your Small Intestine—as felt *through* your Small Intestine. Pretty neat, huh?

The Energy-Cultivating Responses for the Fire Element include satisfaction, joy, enthusiasm, authenticity, and especially love energy. In the Heart is where the magic of life begins. Of all your organs, the Heart is the only one that never gets an hour's rest. So naturally, this makes it very special and worthy of daily appreciation. In fact, your Heart has more Mitochondria per cell than any other organ in the body, with the possible exception of your eyes—and with good reason. Heartbeats take a lot of energy, and fortunately, the cells of your Heart are designed to accommodate this demand for ATP. What's also interesting is that in the East, the eyes are considered the windows to the spirit, and the Heart is where the spirit lives.

The lesson of the Heart is to give it what it needs to produce energy so that it can take care of you in return. Your Heart is a wonderful teacher when it comes to reciprocity—what you do for it, it will do for you. Appreciating your heart for what it gives is an excellent daily habit. Cardiovascular exercise is an act of appreciation. Taking enzyme Coenzyme Q10 (CoQ10) is a wonderful act of appreciation. Simply saying "thank you" is yet another way to show appreciation, and one that sets the stage for all the Energy-Cultivating Responses to reach their maximum effectiveness.

And When Things Go Wrong

I have asked this question of thousands of people in the last decade: What did you immediately feel when you realized you lost a love? Most people will say that they felt sad, angry, or depressed. Having been a veteran of the loss of love myself, I usually tell them that they probably felt something else first. Most people can attest to what I am about to say next. The first thing you felt when love was lost was not anger, frustration, or sadness—although these secondary reactions, or coping mechanisms, probably came shortly afterward. The first thing you probably felt was pain. We don't have a word in our culture that adequately describes this sensation, so I call it Love Pain. Love Pain is an Energy-Draining Reaction, and it can be intense, dramatic, devastating, and paralyzing all at the same time.

It does not matter whether you are a little girl whose father didn't give you enough attention when you deserved it. It doesn't matter if you were a boy who never received his mother's approval. The sensation is still Love Pain. It doesn't matter if you were in a relationship with a boyfriend or girlfriend, or whether you were going through a difficult divorce—the sensation is still Love Pain. If you've watched as a loved one passed away, or if you've ever received a phone call about a family tragedy, you first felt Love Pain. Remember that your body operates on the principle of Sophisticated Simplicity—love unites us, and so does Love Pain. Love Pain it is what we feel first after the loss of love because it is the counterbalance in this world of relativity that we reside in.

It is important to understand that what comes next is part of the perfection of life, even if it doesn't feel good. What often comes next—as it probably should—is the use of secondary-reaction coping mechanisms as we sort through emotional rubble and begin working to rebuild our energy fields and life. In order to heal, it's important to understand What's Good about Love Pain. The **Principle of Advanced Natural Medicine #23** is: *Love Pain is a measurement of how much we really loved. The more it hurts, the more we loved—and that says something very special about us.*

So where will Love Pain take us? Our secondary reactions will be determined by the experience itself and how we choose to cope with it. So long as this is relatively short lived, little to no harm is done to your body. Your body was designed to withstand these temporary life experiences. The problem begins, however, when choosing to keep the Heart closed and the body numb both become a way of life.

As it pertains to the Fire Element, Love Pain can develop into a sense of unworthiness or a sense that we are unworthy of joy, love, happiness, and even good luck. If this false belief is accepted as truth and is also internalized, then the stage is set for degeneration into a third-level reaction known as a behavioral adaptation. At this level of degeneration, it is possible for a person to become very resistant to change, and to easily accept defeat. By the time life has become a series of third-level reactions, the performance of the Heart, Small Intestine, and Thymus are affected. Usually at this point, a decision is made to Change It. Otherwise, a person then begins to experience fourth-level reactions that include self-destructive thought processes, which can seem to provide a sense of safety but actually cause physical harm. At this point, it is very difficult to create the happiness that is necessary to power Mitochondrial Energy Production. Life gets a little worse, and the choice too often is made to slip into the darkness of fifth-level reactions, which include chron-

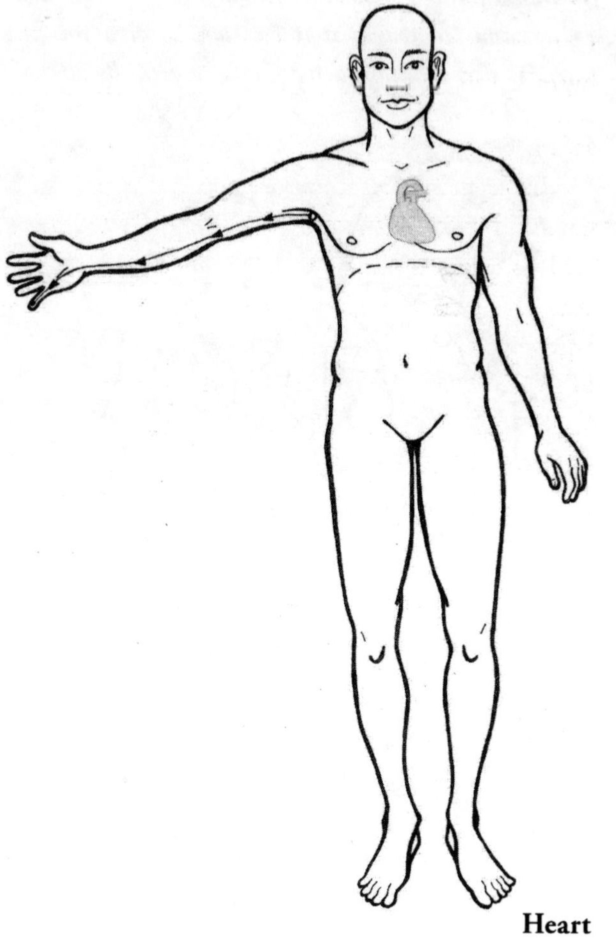

Heart

ic negative internal dialogue and judgment toward self and others. With fifth-level reactions, it is safe to say that physical damage to the Heart, Small Intestine, Thymus, and other organs and glands has already occurred. However, this is also a stage where the potential for healing can be remarkable and exciting.

Additional Associations

The strength of the Heart can be heard in the voice. A voice that cracks, sounds uncertain, or sounds higher pitched than normal or expected can reveal energy disruptions within the Heart. Understand that most problems begin in the energy fields of the body, known as meridians and Chakras. There have been many times when a patient's lab results come back normal, but the patient still feels that something is off or not quite right. *This is a sign of energy disruption, and if not addressed, it eventually will show up in the physical body. Recall the Cycle of Influencing Energy®—Energetics influences emotion, which influences Anatomy-structure, Physiology-organ function, and Biochemistry-cellular energy production. So it stands to reason that emotion is often the first warning sign that something is off energetically.*

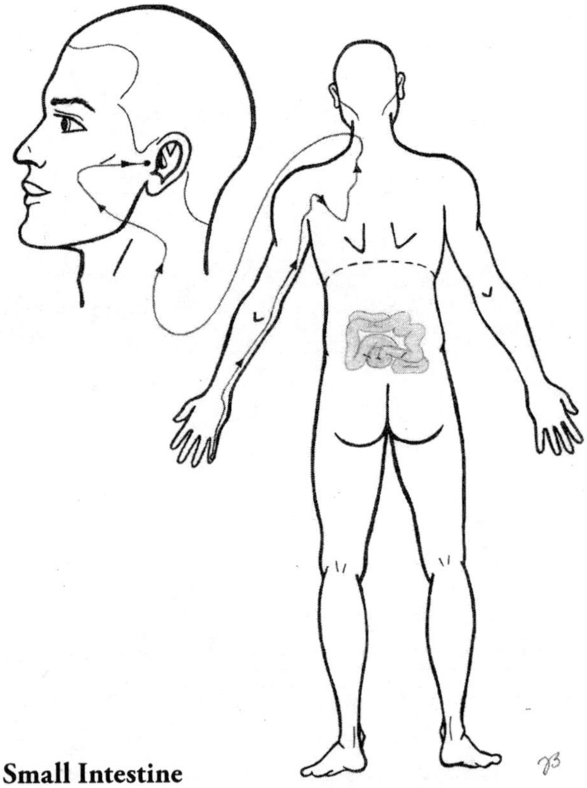

Small Intestine

The health of the Fire Element organs and glands also can be witnessed in the strength and pliability of the blood vessels. People who bruise easily have weak and fragile blood vessels. If blood vessels are weak and fragile, it is usually a sign that the Heart, Small Intestine, and Thymus are likely deficient in some very essential nutrients.

The Heart is most energetically active between 11 A.M. and 1 P.M., while the Small Intestine is most active between 1 P.M. and 3 P.M. This means that our ability to absorb nutrients is greatest between 1 P.M. and 3 P.M. As a result, this is a strong argument for eating the largest meal of the day in the morning or early afternoon for optimal assimilation of nutrients. If you are practicing a Calorie-Restricted Lifestyle, then you might want to have your main meal during this timeframe.

The Fire Element and the affected organs and glands are stimulated by bitter flavors. Bitter flavors encourage enzyme production, which is an essential factor in digestion, detoxification, and immune function.

Energetics: Fire Element Example

Let's consider this example to illustrate this concept. Imagine that a close friend of yours routinely refuses compliments, seldom smiles, and has to be forced to go out for fun. She bruises easily, seldom sweats, rarely works out, and has a difficult time getting to sleep because her thoughts keep her awake.

Which Organs Are Involved?

1. Refuses Compliments—Unworthiness. **Heart, Small Intestine, Thymus**
2. Seldom Smiles—No Joy. **Heart, Small Intestine, Thymus**
3. Has to Be Forced to Go Out—Resistant to Change. **Heart, Small Intestine, Thymus**
4. Bruises Easily, Seldom Sweats. **Heart, Small Intestine, Thymus**
5. Can't Stop Thinking—Mental Chatter. **Spleen-Pancreas, Stomach, Adrenals**

Energetics: Earth Element

Yin Organ	Spleen-Pancreas
Yang Organ	Stomach
Gland	Pancreas
Energetic Associations	Smooth Muscle—Think Tubes Like Digestive Tract
Fluids	Saliva
Tissues	Skeletal Muscles
Time	Spleen-Pancreas 9A.M.–11 A.M., Stomach 7 A.M.–9 A.M.
Flavor	Sweet
Energy-Draining Reactions	Excessive Concentration, Busy, Overwhelmed
Energy-Cultivating Responses	Rational Decision-Making, Clear and Calm Mind

What's Interesting?

The flavor that stimulates digestion is sweet. When we choose sweets that naturally occur in nature like nutrient-dense Organic fruits, vegetables, and grains, they tend to balance our moods, which leads to rational decision making—thanks in part to a clear and calm mind. When we choose empty-calorie, nutrient-deficient, and over-sweetened sodas, candies, and energy drinks, Acidic Cellular Environments often result. And these Acidic Cellular Environments tend to lead to emotional imbalances, which often are experienced as overwhelmed feelings, incessant mental chatter, and insomnia.

Life Lessons for Energy Cultivation

Energy cultivation in life is about creating momentum. One good decision can lead to another, and that decision can lead to another, and so on. Good decision-making is the key to creating momentum in life. Possessing a clear, calm mind greatly assists rational decision-making, and this creates positive momentum. A clean body makes for a clear mind. Keep this in mind when you are learning about the Wood Element.

So obviously, this element has a great deal to do with digestion, thanks in part to the Spleen-Pancreas and the Stomach. Is it better to eat fast-food meals driving alone at 40-plus miles an hour in a rush to get to some destination? Or is it better to eat Organic meals prepared at home with friends and family as a way to celebrate the day? I wonder which choice best supports the clear and calm mind needed for rational, momentum-building decision-making? Just a thought.

And When Things Go Wrong

The Earth Element consists of the Spleen-Pancreas and the Stomach. We group the Spleen and the Pancreas together based on the similarity of their function between Western and Eastern Medicines—even though these two organs are not grouped together in Traditional Chinese Medicine. The Energy-Draining Reaction that most depletes Spleen-Pancreas energy is excessive concentration. This phenomenon is common for disciplined students, doctors, accountants, engineers, computer programmers, and any profession that requires long hours of uninterrupted concentration. Excessive concentration leads to mental exhaustion, fatigue, and ultimately, poor decision-making.

What does excessive concentration lead to but a sense of being busy? In modern times, this may be one of our greatest obstacles to cure—that we are simply doing too many things. We spend too much time on the go, and not enough time on being still. It's as though we are always on emotional overdrive—a situation that leads to feeling drained and empty. It is curious that we overuse our minds after long days of concentration, and then we expect them to turn off like light switches when we decide to go to sleep.

When our mental energy is depleted, but our task list grows, the natural degenerative progression is the sense of being overwhelmed. So how do you know when enough is enough, and that it's time to recharge the batteries? Are you ready for this? When practicing Energy-Cultivating Responses becomes an effort, and it feels more satisfying to use Energy-Draining Reactions. If expressing anger feels satisfying, then you probably have too much on your plate, and likely need a break.

What's more, when practicing Energy-Cultivating Responses becomes an effort they lose their authentic quality and can easily lead to avoidance and resentment.

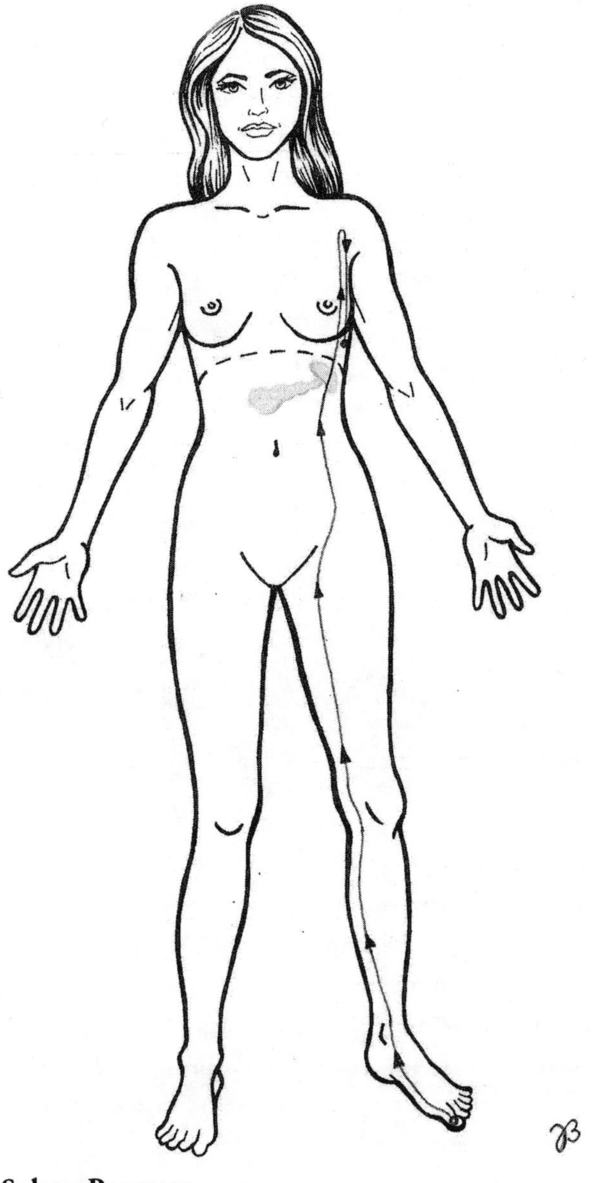

Spleen-Pancreas

Have you ever overcommitted yourself and looked forward to a weekend off, only to realize that you promised to help someone? What did you feel? Perhaps you felt a slight resentment inside and struggled with honoring your commitment. Perhaps you considered making up an excuse to get out of the commitment. If your thoughts are negative or you are thinking of making up excuses, then what are you really saying to yourself? Perhaps it's as simple as realizing that you are out of balance, overwhelmed, and that you need time to enjoy life at a slower pace for awhile.

If you understand the experience of feeling overwhelmed, then perhaps you are willing to deepen your understanding further and consider the effects on your digestion. Remember that there is no difference between the emotion and the effect it has on the body. In this case, feeling overwhelmed results in the activation of the Fight-or-Flight Nervous System, and the shutdown of digestive enzyme production. A person who is stressed out and easily overwhelmed is effectively turning off his or her digestion system because the part of their Nervous System that governs digestion is turned off. Try digesting a meal while you're stressed out. Does feeling tied in knots ring a bell?

Simplification is the solution. Change It by simplifying it. The **Principle of Advanced Natural Medicine #24** is: *Make life as easy as possible—Think Simple.* A to-do list that has more than four or five things to accomplish in a typical day is too long, unrealistic, and it sets you up for failure. Limit yourself and simplify. The reality is that anything more than those four or five things is going to drain your Spleen-Pancreas energy. After you have accomplished those four or five things on your list, you can either continue working to accomplish more tasks if your energy is strong, or you can simply be satisfied with your accomplishments, and give yourself some encouragement and a Mental High Five. What's so bad about enjoying the rest of your day, your family and friends, and getting ready for tomorrow? Your digestive system will be grateful.

Understand too that rest is a good decision, which in turn, helps create many more good decisions. Rest is essential for creating positive momentum in your life.

Additional Associations

During meditation, practitioners often begin to salivate while breathing. Salivation is a sign that the Rest-and-Digest Nervous System is engaged, and that the organs and glands of the Earth Element are being replenished. The Rest-and-Digest Nervous System counterbalances the Fight-or-Flight Nervous System, and is an essential component of all Healing Processes.

The Rest-and-Digest Nervous System rules smooth muscles. Smooth muscles can be found anywhere in the body where there is a tube, such as the digestive tract or blood vessels. Smooth muscles are under the control of the Rest-and-Digest division of the Autonomic Nervous System and influenced by the health of and energy flow from the Spleen-Pancreas and Stomach. Tension in these muscles inhibit their function and are common cofactors of digestive diseases and high blood pressure, which is also known as hypertension.

The health of skeletal muscles—like biceps and quadriceps—is influenced by the health of the Digestive System, and specifically, the energy that flows from the Spleen-Pancreas and the Stomach. Difficulty maintaining muscle mass can be a sign that there are problems in these digestive organs.

The Stomach is at its peak energetic performance between 7 A.M. and 9 A.M., while the Spleen-Pancreas is at its peak energetic performance between 9 A.M. and 11 A.M. Because the Small Intestine's peak energetic performance is between 1 P.M. and 3 P.M., this lends strong credence to the practice of eating the largest meal of the day when the digestive energy is at its peak. Strongly consider adopting the habit of eating the largest meal of your day before 3 P.M. if your schedule allows such flexibility.

Energetics: Earth Element Example

Your family member tells you that he often eats while driving, but lately he notices that the food seems to sit there. He says that his work responsibilities are increasing and he doesn't have enough time in the day to get everything done. He notes that he is getting little colds more frequently, and that he is having trouble getting to sleep because he can't stop thinking about work the next day.

Which Organs Are Involved?

1. Food Seems to Sit—Poor Digestion.
   Spleen-Pancreas, Stomach

2. Not Enough Time—Overwhelmed.
   Spleen-Pancreas, Stomach

3. Frequent Colds—Deficient Immune System.
   Lungs, Large Intestine, Thyroid

4. Can't Stop Thinking—Mental Chatter.
   Spleen-Pancreas, Stomach, Adrenals

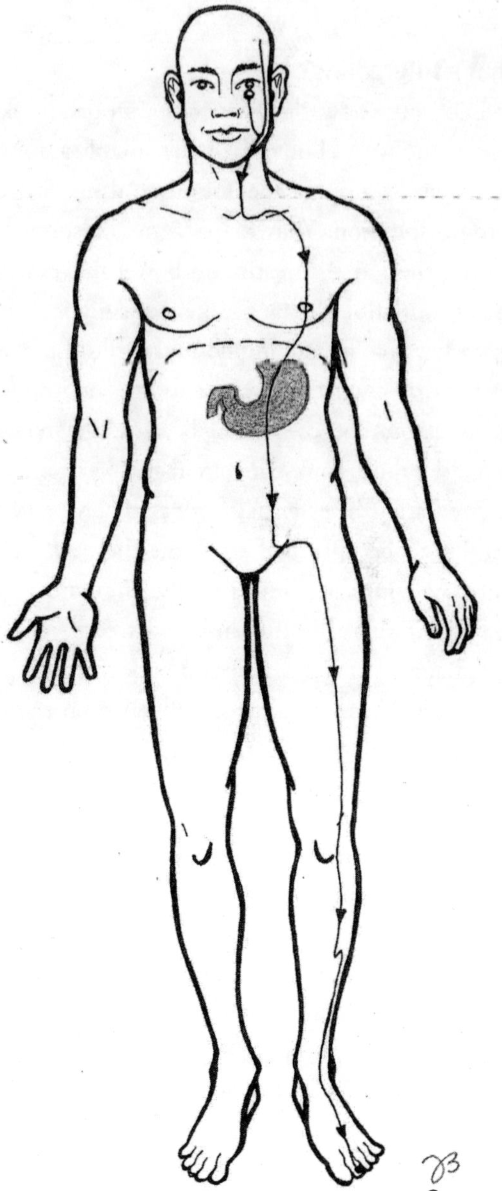

Stomach

Energetics: Gold Element

Yin Organ	Lungs
Yang Organ	Large Intestine
Gland	Thyroid, Parathyroid
Energetic Associations	Immune Cells
Fluids	Lymph
Tissues	Skin, Lymph Nodes
Time	Lungs 3 A.M. – 5 A.M., Large Intestine 5 A.M. – 7 A.M.
Flavor	Hot and Spicy (Pungent)
Energy-Draining Reactions	Grief, Keeping It Locked Inside, Can't Let Go
Energy-Cultivating Responses	Forgiving, Truthful, Encouraging, Positive Communication

What's Interesting?

Did you know that the most important skeletal muscle in your body is your diaphragm? Your diaphragm is responsible for expanding the Lungs during inspiration. Your diaphragm is responsible for assisting the Large Intestine in bowel movement and waste elimination. What's more, your diaphragm also plays a key role in moving lymphatic fluid upward so that it can reenter blood circulation. The importance of this cannot be overstated because the reentry of lymphatic fluid into the circulatory system allows the circulation of essential fatty acids and fat-soluble vitamins to be absorbed from the diet. As well, the reentry of lymphatic fluid into the circulatory system releases immune cells into the bloodstream. As a result, your diaphragm—the major muscle responsible for respiration—has a significant influence on the health of your Immune System, the Gold Element, and all of its Energetic associations.

Life Lessons for Energy Cultivation

The Energetics of the Gold Element has a great deal to do with communication. After the healing decision has been made and healing skills have been instituted, the primary healing responses for the Gold Element include truthfulness, continued encouragement, and their offspring—positive communication with everyone you meet. I can appreciate any doubt you might have toward that last part of the sentence—everyone you meet. You may be thinking of someone who you feel you simply cannot communicate positively with. To that I would respond: Are you more concerned about the outcome of the interaction, or how you participate in it? When you give yourself the freedom to be more concerned about your participation than the outcome, you can cultivate inner satisfaction from your participation. By making the interaction about your energy production and the satisfaction that can result from that, there is no logical reason for you to have less than positive communication with everyone you meet. Positive communication is in your best interest.

The secret is that this has always been about you, and always will be about you. Inherent in this truth is ultimate freedom. This concept is not selfish, but rather benevolent, as it engages a deep sense of personal integrity and accountability for your actions and your actions alone. So now let's apply this potentially difficult concept to the art of forgiveness. Yes—it is an art, not an obligation. Forgiveness works best as an art when it is practiced from a genuine place of authenticity. This translates to the belief that forgiveness should never be forced or fake. Forgiveness happens when you are ready to forgive completely from your heart, and not a moment before. But herein lies another secret that is based on the first idea in this paragraph: Every moment you decide against forgiveness is a moment you and your body have to carry the burden. The longer you decide to carry the burden, the heavier it becomes. This can set you up for entering into third-, fourth-, and fifth-level Energy-Draining Reactions. The choice of letting go of your troubles is yours and always has been. The art of forgiveness is the art of letting go, and avoiding the temptation of becoming a victim. To forgive is to let go. To have the ability to let go is to consistently focus more on your actions than on the actions of others—especially those that offend you. Just a thought.

And When Things Go Wrong

The predominant Energy-Draining Reaction in the Gold Element is the experience of grief. Grief is very interesting because it is a prolonged sadness—a grieving process—that is part of the healing. One afternoon, I was listening to Dr. Gladys McGarey lecture, and as she often does, she said something quite profound. She said: "There is no pill for grief, the medicine is time and expression." Too often, the feeling of sadness is valid, but has not been adequately expressed to the grieving person's satisfaction. As a result, there is a tendency to hold onto it and lock it into the body. Laugh out loud, and the whole world laughs with you; cry, and you cry alone.

When you make a choice to internalize what you feel, you simultaneously interrupt the grieving process and lock everything you are feeling into your body's Nervous System. Expression is a key component of the grieving process. At first, the decision to internalize sadness typically begins to show up as changes in eating and sleeping patterns. Eventually, however, this can begin to have a more drastic impact on your body's anatomical structure. It begins to affect how you stand, walk, sit, and especially how you breathe. Remember from the Cycle of Influencing Energy® that emotion is going to influence Anatomy, so when I see people walking down the street with their chest sunken in and their shoulders sloped forward, I know that their Gold Element Lung energy is weak. I know that the person's Heart is retracted, revealing Love Pain that is showing up as a secondary reaction of internalized sadness. So in applying Energetic thought, I know that there are two major organs involved—their Heart due to Love Pain, and their Lungs as a result of grief. Words can be deceiving, but the body does not know how to lie if you know its language. And certainly, posture is a major language of the body. The **Principle of Advanced Natural Medicine #25** is: *Your body does not know how to lie—in your body lives only the truth.*

Understand that Love Pain can't remain present in a person's life day after day after day. So a choice is often made to 'put it away,' or internalize, the Love Pain. When Love Pain is internalized, it results in a secondary reaction that is used to cope with the situation. It also leads to an overload on the Nervous System, which has a numbing effect. It is for this reason that many people who have internalized Love Pain have a difficult time feeling anything good, bad, or otherwise. In fact, some people welcome the numbness because even that can be an improvement from the Love Pain. As mentioned earlier, a secondary reaction can be a healthy and quite normal aspect of the Healing Process. But it is cause for concern when the secondary reaction is prolonged, leading to behavioral adaptations and the eventual downward spiral into third-, fourth-, and fifth-level Energy-Draining Reactions.

Of all the Energy-Draining Reactions, grief is the most concerning because it is a very low energy state to begin with, and it can be very difficult to overcome if a person begins to isolate and becomes sedentary. Does grief affect how a person breathes? Absolutely. Let's explore that.

I'd like you to sit up straight with both feet on the floor. Next, lean forward and hug yourself. Now, take the biggest breath you can take. This mimics the anatomical effect that a sunken chest has on your breath. Now, sit up straight again and place your hands on your thighs. Activate your feet, and feel your spine extending upward as you breathe in. Compare the two breaths—which one was larger and easier?

Obviously the second breath. So does emotion have the ability to influence Anatomy? Yes, indeed. A person who has a sunken chest has to work harder just to breathe. They have to work harder to get oxygen to their cells, and as a result, this places a huge burden on their Heart, which then has to pump faster and work harder. *The reason posture is so important—and why Yoga Therapy stresses it so much—is because posture greatly influences how we breathe. The more aligned the posture, the easier it is to breathe, and for every organ in the body to function.*

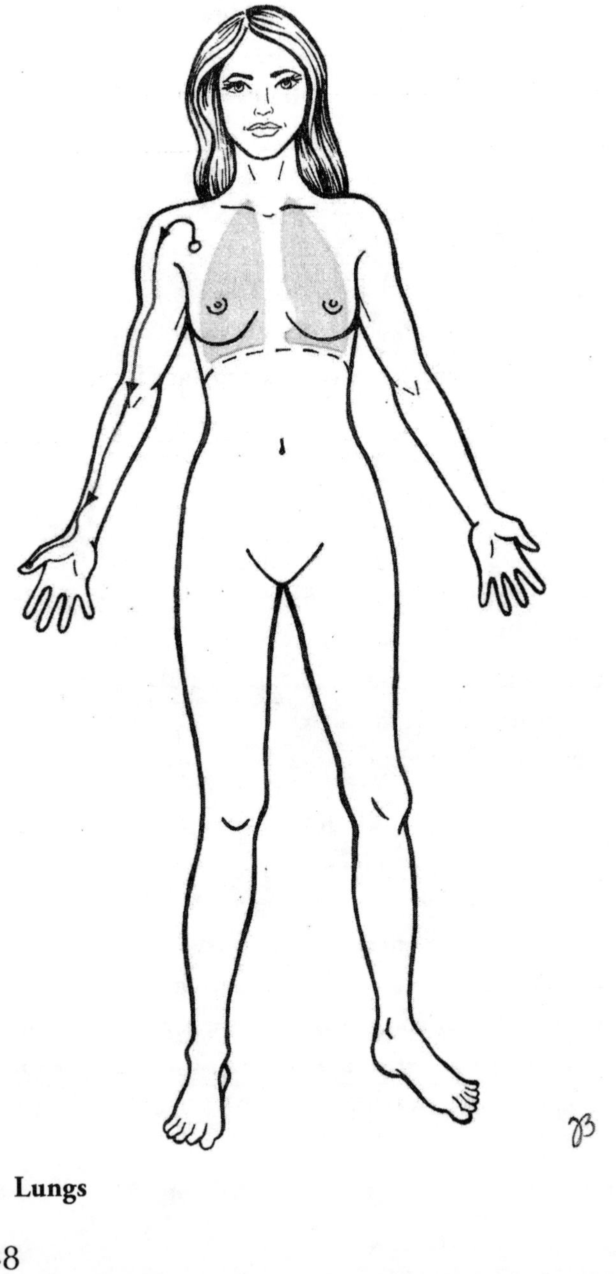

Lungs

When applying the lessons of the Gold Energetics, know that you can hold onto whatever you want, for as long as you want. Just keep in mind that the longer you hold onto whatever *it* is, the heavier *it* is going to get for you and your body. When you are ready to let it go, Change It. Hopefully, your response will include forgiveness somewhere in there. When you are ready in your Heart to forgive whoever it is who hurt you, something magical will happen—*your body will feel lighter*. That sense of feeling lighter in your body is the undeniable reality that you have let go, and that you are no longer letting it affect your life.

How do you know when you have healed through the art of forgiveness? Great question! You know that you have healed using the art of forgiveness when you can recount whatever the circumstance was without losing energy or looking for sympathy as a victim. Very rarely will I allow myself or one of my patients to play victim—it is a seductive way to get lost in the disease process. One of my favorite things to listen for in conversation is humorous resiliency when a person recounts a challenging story. You will know that you have forgiven from your Heart, and that you have healed as a result when your body feels lighter. You won't feel any loss of energy when you think about the circumstance, and especially when you can recall the event with a sense of humor. Obviously, not all events will have a humorous aspect, but we will discuss this more in future volumes.

The Lungs are at their energetic peak between 3 A.M. and 5 A.M., while the Large Intestine is at its energetic peak between 5 A.M. and 7 A.M. This reveals two interesting insights:

1. When a person frequently wakes between 3 A.M. and 5 A.M., it can reveal a Lung disharmony that potentially has to do with grief and internalized emotions.

2. Since the Large Intestine has its Energetic peak between 5 A.M. and 7 A.M., the best thing you can do upon waking is have a bowel movement.

The Gold Element is associated with the Immune System and the house of the Immune System—the Lymphatic Vessels. Thus, the health of the Lungs and Large Intestine have a HUGE influence over the health of the Immune System. These two organs of the Gold Element, in addition to the Liver, also influence the health of the Skin.

The Gold Element is stimulated by hot and spicy flavors. When a person consumes hot and spicy flavors, the Lungs are able to better distribute energy throughout the body. It is interesting that hot and spicy flavors have the effect of dilating blood vessels so that nutrients can be better distributed to the cellular level.

As a final thought, the Gold Element also includes the Thyroid and Parathyroid Gland. I have long wondered why women have a highly disproportionate number of hypothyroid conditions compared to men. Using Energetics an explanation may provide some insight. Men have a tendency to express themselves to their level of satisfaction, more so than their female counterparts. When a woman has too much on her mind and keeps it inside, the act of keeping it inside often becomes a contributing factor in the development of hypothyroidism.

Energetics: Gold Element Example

You come home and notice your mother washing dishes after a long day of work. She appears frustrated, but you ask her what's wrong she says with a forced smile, "Everything's fine." She has been diagnosed with Hypothyroidism, and was improperly taught that healthy bowel movements occur only once per week, which she proudly never discusses. She is pleasing to a fault, and seldom says what is on her mind. Instead, she prefers to change the subject or ignore the question when she is uncomfortable. She also typically wakes up around 3:30 A.M. every morning and has a difficult time getting back to sleep.

Which Organs Are Involved?

1. Frustrated. **Liver, Gallbladder**
2. False Smile—Keeping It Locked Inside. **Lungs, Large Intestine, Thyroid**
3. Hypothyroidism. **Lungs, Large Intestine, Thyroid**
4. Constipation. **Lungs, Large Intestine, Thyroid**
5. Pleasing to a Fault—Internalization. **Lungs, Large Intestine, Thyroid**
6. Doesn't Discuss What Is On Her Mind. **Lungs, Large Intestine, Thyroid**
7. Wakes up at 3:30 A.M.—**Lung Time. Lungs, Large Intestine, Thyroid**

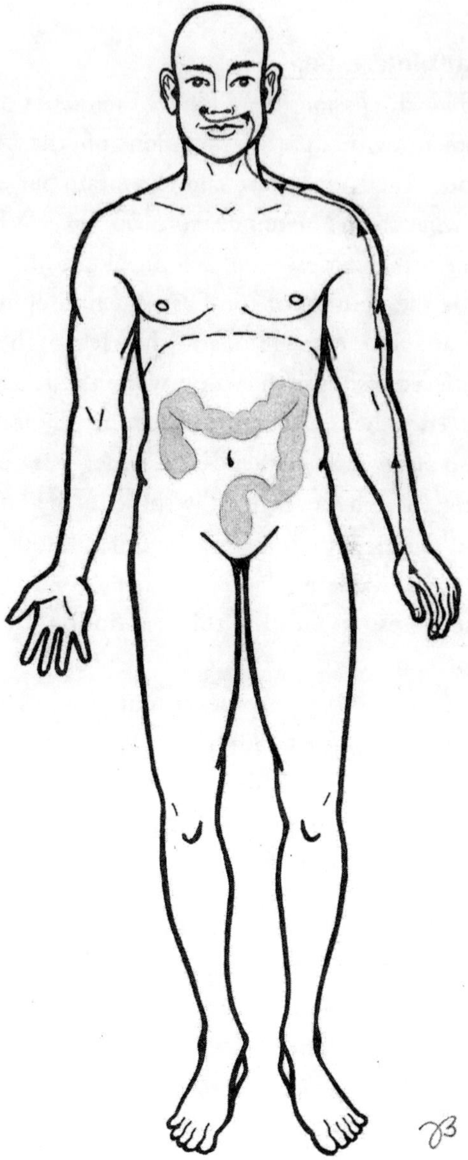

Large Intestine

Energetics: Water Element

Yin Organ	Kidneys
Yang Organ	Urinary Bladder
Gland	Adrenal and Reproductive
Energetic Associations	Ears and Head Hair
Fluids	Urine, Semen
Tissues	Bones
Time	Kidneys 5 P.M. – 7 P.M., Urinary Bladder 3 P.M. – 5 P.M.
Flavor	Salty
Energy-Draining Reactions	Lack of Trust, Fear, Worry, Anxiety
Energy-Cultivating Responses	Trusting in Life's Perfection, Faithful, Belief

What's Interesting?

No discussion of Kidney Energetics can be complete without the inclusion of the Adrenal Glands. The Kidneys are said to contain our essence, also what the Chinese refer to as our *Jing*. While the Kidneys play an essential role in blood filtration, it also is the opinion of the Eastern philosophies that they are close companions to the Heart. The Heart is believed to house the spirit, while the Kidneys are believed to be the foundation for the physical body. It also believed that when Kidney energy is no longer strong enough to anchor the spirit to the body, the spirit passes into the next lifetime. Quite poetic, really. In Western Physiology, the Adrenal Glands come closest to meeting this description, thanks to a hormone they secrete called Cortisol. Cortisol, for all intents and purposes, is our physical essence. Without it, Mitochondria cannot produce energy, and without energy, life as we know it ceases. This is the energetic connection between the Kidneys and the Adrenal Glands.

Life Lessons for Energy Cultivation.

Having the belief that you will heal essentially nourishes your body with that emotion. The **Principle of Advanced Natural Medicine #26** is: *Belief is as essential to a Healing Process as any natural medicine.* Belief is a beautiful, inexpensive medicine. What you choose to practice emotionally affects the cells of that particular organ. When you nourish the cells of a particular organ, it improves the function of that organ, the entire organ system, and the entire body. In this particular example, when you practice belief, you are improving how your Kidneys clean your blood so that your cells can receive nutrient-dense blood that is free of waste matter.

I am always reminded of a press conference held by Ervin "Magic" Johnson in late 1991. During his press conference, Magic came out before the world and announced that he had contracted HIV. We all have moments in life when we can recall where we were when something historic or tragic happened. I've heard family members talk about where they were when Martin Luther King and Malcolm X were murdered. I've heard more people than I can count tell me stories of where they were when President Kennedy and his brother were assassinated. In every situation, each person mentioned feeling a loss of hope, and a loss in belief. When Magic announced he had contracted HIV, it was believed at that time that HIV was a death sentence. There was a tremendous amount of fear about this new killer. And during his press conference, Magic said something I'll never forget. He said, "I know that God gave me this disease because he knew I could beat it."

At the time of this press conference, I was attending the University of California, Los Angeles and was glued to the TV with all of my fellow Lakers friends. We all thought he was courageous. We all thought he was brave for saying what he did. But we did not believe he was going to overcome the disease. Yet nearly twenty years later, Magic lives. From day one, he told the world about his belief, and then he took action and learned everything he could to support that belief in his abilities. Regardless of the outcome, he won by believing. How wonderful is it that he's still with us? It's amazing what we can do when we believe.

I've heard through the grapevine that Magic immediately began paying strict attention to his diet, and even endorsed a brand of medicinal mushrooms noted for their ability to boost the Immune System. His decisions created clean alkaline blood in his body, and that gave his Immune System a chance to fight. Understand that the cleaner the blood, the better the Mitochondrial Energy cultivation, and as a result, the better the immune response. Remember, when you do one positive thing in the Cycle of Influencing Energy®, it carries itself all the way through the entire cycle. The more things that you add into the mix and the more points of entry that you give yourself—through Energy-Cultivating Responses, Eating Healthy, and great natural therapies—the greater likelihood that energy will synergize and resonate. With healing resonance, the Healing Process will accelerate for you.

So how do you know when you are practicing Energy-Cultivating Responses for your Water Element? Whenever you are practicing belief, faithfulness, and trust you are supporting Mitochondrial Energy Production within the Kidneys, Urinary Bladder, Reproductive Glands, and Adrenal Glands.

The Kidneys have everything to do with trust. We trust that our Heart is going to beat without fail each day. We trust that our Digestive System will perform well with each meal. We trust that literally trillions of biochemical transformations will occur at the cellular level every blink of an eye, and in every moment of our lives. Trust is an essential part of our lives, and it is something we engage in with every breath—even when we fail to appropriately show our appreciation for the beauty we are so fortunate to experience each day. To be able to breathe is beautiful, in and of itself. So when was the last time you told your body how much you appreciate it for doing its job day in and day out? Today's a good day for that. In fact, there's no time like the present. Give props to your body, then give yourself a Mental High Five.

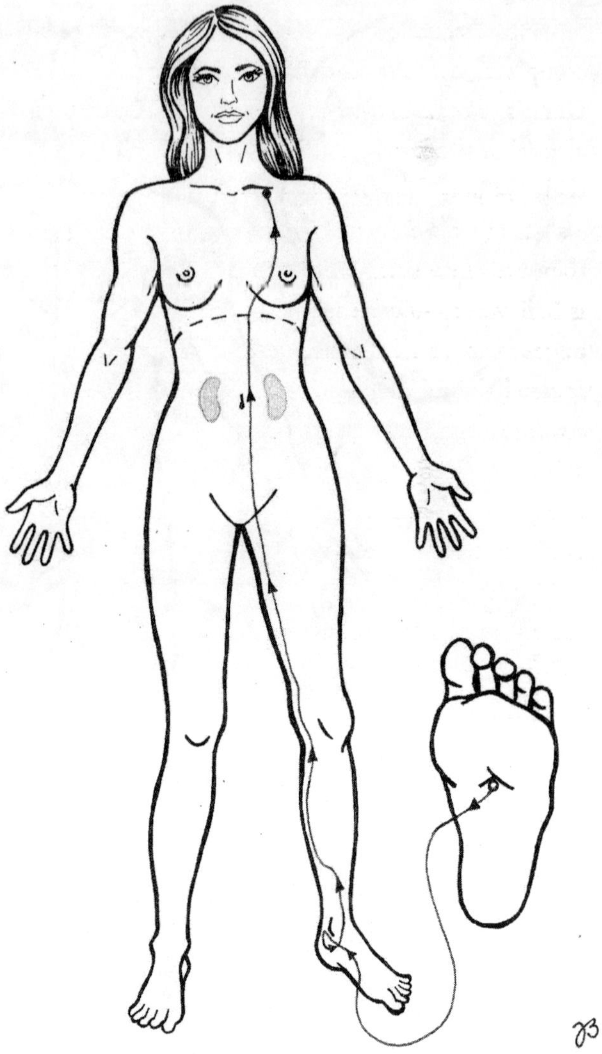

Kidneys

And When Things Go Wrong

So much of what we know about life is based on trust. The adverse effects on the body become quite clear when we deliberately break the trust essential for living at ease. Traditionally, the concept of Water Element Energetics is taught to encompass fear, anxiety, doubt, and worry. What are those Energy-Draining Reactions, but the result of a lack of trust. A loss of trust in life's perfection is what happens before a person gets worried, anxious, and/or fearful. Thus, the classic Energy-Draining Reactions are actually third-level behavioral adaptations resulting from a lack of trust. When a person is consumed by fear, and bases decision-making on this illusion, the logical outcome is for that person to seek ways to control what is going on in every aspect of life. What a tremendous toll this way of thinking has on the Adrenal Glands, Cortisol levels, Mitochondrial Energy Production and the entire body.

The desire for a certain amount of control is completely understandable, so long as it is not based in fear. It's difficult to imagine a parent who has no desire to establish boundaries for their growing children. For many people, life has led to Love Pain, along with questioning about why the circumstance involving the Love Pain happened. Without a secure, rational answer, many of these same people decide to take matters into their own hands so that they do not have to feel that Love Pain again.

It's okay to fall down. It's okay to get hurt. Love Pain shows us how much we really loved in the first place. It says so many wonderful things about who we are, and also about the experience of being human. Here's a thought for those of you who've experienced Love Pain—we should all be so lucky to experience it many times over during our lifetime. Why? Because that means we have

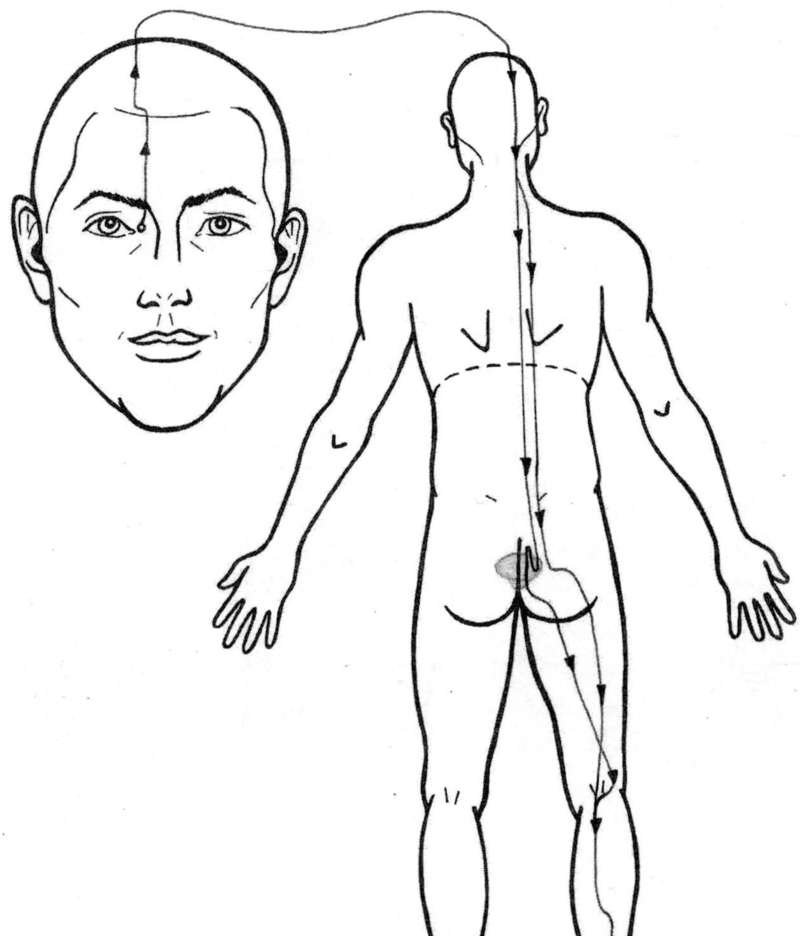

Urinary Bladder

experienced love many times during our lifetime. It means that we were open to the experience, and we continued coming back again and again and again.

With trust permeating our every decision, there is little need to be hypercontrolling. But let's look at this common process in more detail.

We experience Love Pain, and then we begin to engage in healthy secondary reaction coping mechanisms. After a certain amount of time—which is different for everyone and every situation—we decide whether we want to heal again. Is it the correct time to open ourselves back up to experience love energy again? If we need more time, we can't stay in Love Pain because it is too damaging and too hard on the spirit.

Many people will experience a secondary reaction like losing trust in life, themselves, and the people around them. From there, another secondary reaction develops that helps divert their attention away from how they feel. Have you ever felt emotional pain, and then plunged head first into your work? If this is you, for example, then you might begin to engage in excessive concentration as another secondary reaction that depletes the energy of the Earth Element. While doing this, you also might begin to crave sweet foods because your Earth Element is depleted. If you choose candy, sodas, and energy drinks in a vain effort to stimulate your Earth Energetics back into balance, then the result will be the addition of Acidic Cellular Environments, and more stress, damage, and fatigue. When you begin to understand and practice Energetics, you begin to realize that there is a reason for almost everything.

Delving into work can be a way to avoid emotions that don't feel very good, but it also is not a viable long-term solution. If you have had reason to lose trust, it is not outside the realm of possibility that you will find yourself worrying more and more about things that never used to bother you. From lack of trust, to worry, and then to fear—this is the common path of unresolved and internalized Love Pain. And if something is avoided, it usually gets worse.

Without trust, hypercontrolling habits sometimes result in further disconnecting you from the real root of the problem. The root of the problem is—and always has been—Love Pain. The root of the problem is that the Heart is hurt, and that the fearful person has never learned the skills necessary to effectively overcome this obstacle to healing. The skill is trust. Trusting is a skill, along with the practice of discernment—which is directly related to the foundation of trust.

I am not suggesting that you trust everyone and everything. But I am suggesting that you trust in life and its perfection. I am suggesting that you trust in the idea that there is something far greater than ourselves at work that is waiting for you to trust its reassuring protection. As you learn to discern what is right and wrong, and what is safe and dangerous—by listening to a clean and open Heart—it will become easier and easier to trust in the perfection of life.

Let's say you know someone who is not very trusting—perhaps even fearful. Let's examine why that behavioral adaptation might have developed.

Lack of trust is typically experienced by a person who has experienced consistent or a large number of negative experiences. Typically one event—even if it is intense—is not enough to create a fearful person. We have someone who got their hopes up. And then when their hopes were dashed, they got back on the horse again, got their hopes up, and then had them trampled again. I wonder how much of this cycle developed in high school, especially around the time that dating started? When a person consistently feels that their hopes are dashed, the person will learn to adapt in the short term. But if the failures inspire more creativity, then they can be a blessing in disguise. However, if a person starts thinking: *I just can't trust that my hopes and dreams are ever going to be realized*, then what develops is uncertainty and fear. *When a person doesn't feel entitled to dream*, life is a very sad, dark place to be.

No one likes to lose, and yet a person who chooses not to dream as a result of previous disappointment has done just that. A person without dreams is lost.

Logically, what can this person do to tip the scales in their favor? One answer is to become hypercontrolling. The problem is the enormous toll this takes on the whole body. And here's a little fact of life: It is a very, very rare person who enjoys the company of a person who is distrustful, fearful, anxious, hypercontrolling, and who is without dreams. Walking around this way is almost a surefire way to remain alone in the world. So what comes next? Sometimes a little negative internal dialogue and judgment—even better ways for a person to alienate himself or herself from others who are close to them. Remember where this all began? Love Pain.

Does this sound like anyone you know? What's so interesting is that we've all practiced Energetics all along without realizing it.

Additional Associations.

Salty is the flavor that stimulates Kidney Energy. So it probably come as no surprise that many people who work too much end up draining their Adrenal Glands and engaging in excessive concentration. This leads to the two most predominant cravings—salty (Water Element), and sweet (Earth Element).

The Kidneys are said to be at their energetic peak between 5 P.M. and 7 P.M., while the Urinary Bladder is said to be at its energetic peak between 3 P.M. and 5 P.M. Truthfully, there is not a tremendous amount of useful information from this observation unless a particular treatment plan is designed to heal the Kidneys. But perhaps it would make sense to dose nutrients or apply therapy during these timeframes.

The Water Element is closely related to the health of the reproductive glands and tissues. Any erectile dysfunction or waning desire for intimacy can be attributed to the Water Element. The reproductive glands and tissues also are related to the Wood Element. While the Water Element has a great deal to do with function and desire, the Wood Element plays a significant role in hormone production and balance.

The tissue associated with the Water Element is bone. For this reason, any history of fragile bones, osteoporosis, or osteopenia is a sign of depleted Kidney Energy. Similarly, persistent ringing of the ears—also known as tinnitus—is a sign of depleted Kidney Energy.

Energetics: Water Element Example

Your father tells you about his younger days and some of the risks he and his friends used to take in their pursuit of fun. So you ask him to tell you about the last time he took a similar risk. And he replies: "Why would I do that now?" Because he had a good time, you tell him. And then he says: "I have more responsibilities now, more things to worry about like paying all these bills." Then he tells you his lower back has been hurting more lately, and that he often wakes up feeling tired. He wonders aloud if any of this might be due to his enlarged prostate.

Which Organs Are Involved?

1. "Why Would I Do That Now? —Lack of Desire. **Kidney, Urinary Bladder, Adrenals**
2. Worried About Paying Bills. **Kidney, Urinary Bladder, Adrenals**
3. Low Back Pain—Deficient Kidney Energy. **Kidney, Urinary Bladder, Adrenals**
4. Waking Tired—Adrenal Fatigue. **Kidney, Urinary Bladder, Adrenals**
5. Enlarged Prostate. **Kidney, Urinary Bladder, Adrenals, Reproductive Glands**

ENERGETICS: WOOD ELEMENT

Yin Organ	Liver
Yang Organ	Gallbladder
Gland	Liver and Reproductive Organs
Energetic Associations	Whites of the Eyes (Sclera), Body Hair, Uterus
Fluids	Tears
Tissues	Ligaments, Tendons, Fascia
Time	Liver 1 A.M. – 3 A.M., Gallbladder 11 P.M. – 3 A.M.
Flavor	Sour
Energy-Draining Reactions	Anger, Mood Instability, Frustration, Complaining, Impatience, Indecisiveness, Timidity, Lack of Confidence
Energy-Cultivating Responses	Patience, Peacefulness, Confidence, Accountability, Taking Action

What's Interesting?

Typically when studying and applying Energetics, there is a tendency to concentrate more on the Yin organ. That is to say, when we examine which organ is more influenced by reactions and responses, there is a tendency to associate the reactions and responses with the Yin organs. In reality, both Yin and Yang organs are affected because of their Energetic connections, but still, this is how it traditionally has been taught and applied. With this in mind, there are certain reactions and responses that are specific to Yang organs, and the Wood Element is a fantastic example of such a case.

The Wood Element has a great deal to do with emotional stability and the promotion of rational decision-making (Earth Element). However, it also has a great deal to do with the ability to select a decision and the confidence necessary to be decisive and steadfast in that decision. What's interesting is that confidence and decisiveness are both attributes of Gallbladder Energetics, and so we will discuss two insights. First, in Energetic thought the Gallbladder consists of both the actual Gallbladder, as well as the Bile Ducts that penetrate the Liver tissue. As a result of this, a person who has had their Gallbladder removed still maintains the foundation of their Gallbladder Energetics through the actual Bile Ducts. Second, I have always found it interesting that Lecithin, a nutrient found in beans and legumes, has a high concentration of Choline. Choline plays several roles in your body. It is an essential component of Acetylcholine, your body's most predominant neurotransmitter. As a result, it plays an important role in confidence and decisiveness. It also plays an important role in the elimination of cholesterol and fat via the Bile Ducts.

So in this case, as with many others, you will learn that many concepts that originated in the East through observation have been validated in the West via Physiology and Biochemistry. Interesting indeed.

Life Lessons for Energy Cultivation.

Of all the elements, the Wood Element is the key to achieving the emotional stability, which in turn, helps maintain patience and peacefulness. In order to create emotional stability, it is important to understand the crucial role the Liver plays in the overall function of the body. Your Liver is responsible for a great many functions. It can synthesize proteins and fats, metabolize and store carbohydrates, all while producing the bile necessary to breakdown fats in the diet and eliminate fat-soluble pollution. Truly, your Liver is a multitalented organ-gland charged with keeping the bloodstream very, very clean.

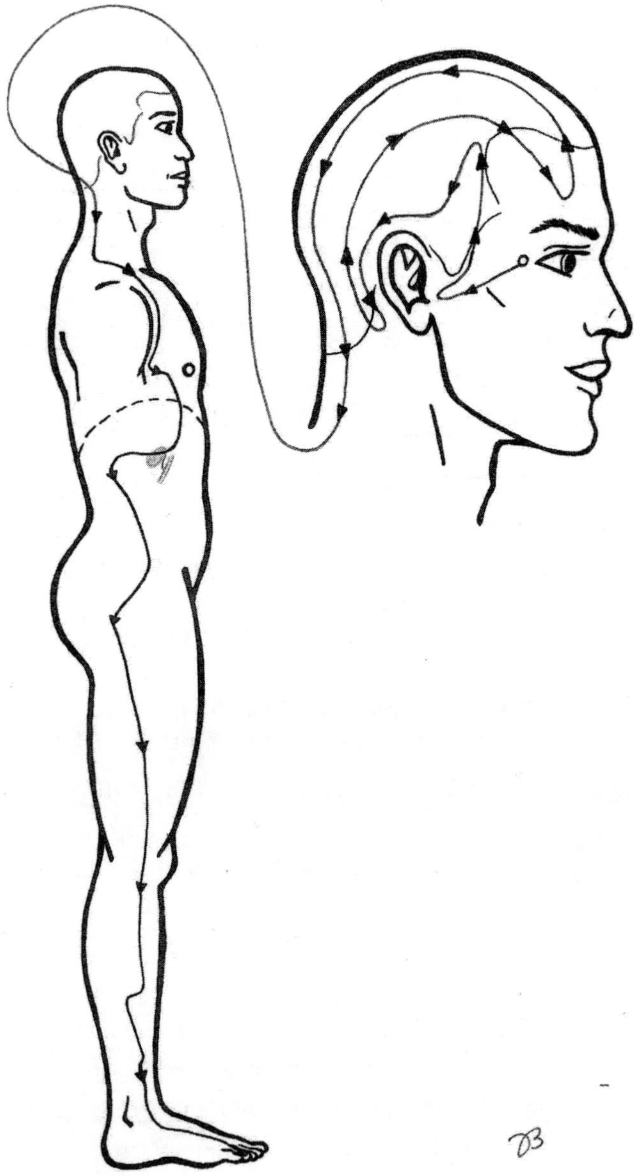

Gallbladder

When you expose yourself to environmental pollutants like chemical air-fresheners, chemical household cleaners, pesticides in produce, and others, your blood gets dirty and that forces your Liver to work harder to clean it up. When you drink alcohol or take recreational drugs, you dirty your blood and force your Liver to work harder to clean it up. Is it any wonder that alcohol and recreational drugs so often result in unstable emotions and poor decision-making? Certainly these should not be considered part of a healthy lifestyle.

The lesson that your emotions provide you is this: The secret to cultivating and maintaining patience, peacefulness, confidence, and decisiveness is a healthy Liver and Gallbladder. Perhaps the best daily gift you can give your Liver and Gallbladder is the gift of clean blood so they don't have to work so hard to clean it up. When you practice Eating Healthy and Energy-Cultivating Responses, you do exactly that—you give your Liver a well-deserved break, and you set the stage for mood stability.

And When Things Go Wrong

At some point in life, we have all been frustrated with things that are out of our control. In today's fast-paced lifestyle, frustration seems to be one of the most common Energy-Draining Reactions.

Frustration directly affects your Liver. And any stress that impacts your Liver can set the stage for frustration. It's Friday night, and the gang's all going out for happy hour. Midway through drink #1, you begin to notice that everyone's eyes are getting bloodshot. Because the whites of the eyes reveal the health of the Liver, and because redness is a sign of inflammation, we know damage is occurring to the Liver. After round #2, you decide to go to the bathroom to relieve your bladder, and you notice that your urine is clear. Here's why: Alcohol wipes out B-complex vitamins, most notably Vitamin B1. These are essential to Mitochondrial Energy Production. Time for round #3, and you notice that the eyes are getting a little more red. You also notice that your filter—the one that translates what you're thinking to what you're saying—seemingly have taken the rest of the night off. Outstanding! Now you're saying what's really on your mind, and you're expressing yourself. You're having a grand time, but as you look around the bar, you notice several people who are getting a little more emotional. Some are getting a little loud and unruly, others are getting a little combative, and some seem to be too touchy-feely and teary-eyed. You are witnessing firsthand how damage to the Liver leads to mood instability.

So why do some people react differently than others? Well, I'm glad you asked. The **Principle of Advanced Natural Medicine #27** is: *The only emotion that will ever come out of someone is what's already living within.*

Now it's the morning after. The night was fun, you got home safe (thanks to a designated driver), and your head is spinning and pounding all at the same time. A neighbor decides to get an early start on the household chores, a gardener is outside blowing leaves around, dogs are barking, and kids are screaming. Are you at peace or are you starting to get a little upset and frustrated that everyone is ruining your day? So what set you up for that experience? Damage to your Liver from the night before.

You can also witness the Liver in action in the field of professional athletics. Referring to the 5-Element Perspective chart, notice that the health of the Liver governs the health of fascia and sinews—also known as Tendons and Ligaments. When Tendons and Ligaments are repeatedly damaged due to strains, sprains, or complete ruptures, there is always a question about why.

An athlete who repeatedly experiences muscle tears or pulls, ankle sprains, or ruptured Tendons or Ligaments likely has a congested Liver—often from dirty blood and preexisting damage that's not repairing adequately. Why is it not repairing? Think nutrient deficiencies plus repetitive stress, plus Acidic Cellular Environments, plus a congested Liver. These all add up to repeat injuries.

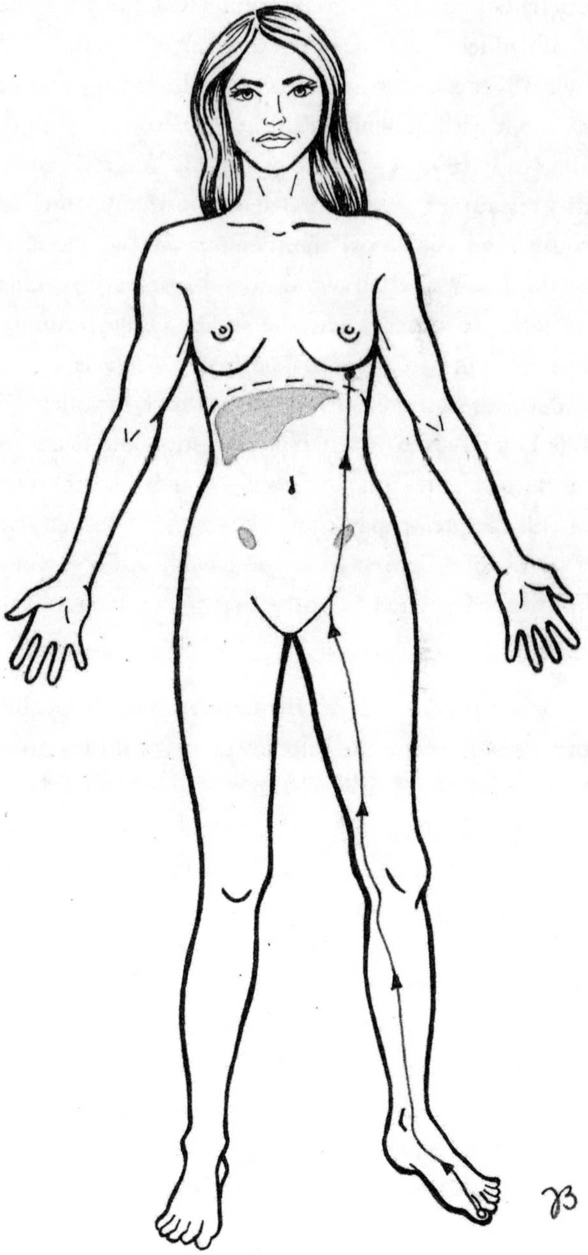

Liver

There are several signs that there is a problem with the Liver, including Energy-Draining Reactions, red eyes, and repetitive injuries to Tendons and Ligaments. Also included in this list are any definitive hormone imbalances. Remember that the Water Element governs the function of the reproductive organs, while Liver Energetics rule the hormonal balance of the reproductive organs.

A discussion of Wood Element Energetics is a great way to demonstrate the distinction between the Yin and Yang organs. But what about Gallbladder Energetics? The Energy-Draining Reactions for the Gallbladder include lack of confidence, timidity, and indecisiveness. Consider this example: Have you ever been out with a friend for dinner, and you are hungry and ready to order a delicious meal? You've been to this restaurant with your friend too many times to count, and you know the menu as well as the chef in the kitchen. BUT, your friend can never decide on what to order when the waiter comes around. Hmmmmm. This is a classic case of indecisiveness and a clear sign the Gallbladder—which includes the Bile Ducts—is experiencing congestion and needs to be flushed out. This last point—much like the rest of this chapter—may sound strange to you because it's probably the first time you have heard how your body is really wired to work. That's okay, keep rolling with it.

Indecisiveness is easily observed when people order from a menu they already know, or if they drive hesitantly, constantly changing lanes, sometimes causing accidents. Indecisiveness also can affect how we choose careers, relationships, investments, and more. A person who is indecisive stifles momentum in their life. As success becomes a hit-or-miss proposition, doubt and lack of confidence often surface, resulting in a person who has problems making up his or her mind and who ends up stuck in indecision. These are the kinds of people who often are taken advantage of, and who are taken for granted. This is a real shame because this all can be turned around with a healthy Gallbladder and some proper skill development.

Additional Associations.

A sour flavor is what stimulated the Wood Element and the Liver and Gallbladder to increase their detoxifying power. It should come as no surprise that lemons have been used to cleanse the Liver for thousands of years.

The Gallbladder is most active between 11 P.M. and 1 A.M., while the Liver is most active energetically between 1 A.M. and 3 A.M. This gives us tremendous insight into the connection between insomnia and Liver health. It is no accident that many people who suffer from insomnia frequently wake up between 1 and 3 A.M. during active Liver time. Certainly we can view insomnia as imbalances in neurotransmitters, including serotonin, dopamine, epinephrine, and norepinephrine. But why are they imbalanced? For the answer, look to the health of the Liver. If a person is going to be able to overcome insomnia, there will have to be improvements made in several areas. But a failure to improve the health of the Liver may lead to inconsistent results.

The Liver and Gallbladder also play instrumental roles in maintaining hormonal balance. Because your Liver is responsible for detoxifying excess hormones, any imbalances or excesses in hormones like estrogen or testosterone can be attributed to an unhappy Liver. While the Liver is responsible for detoxifying excess hormones, the Gallbladder is actually responsible for getting rid of them through the bile. So the two organs work in concert to help balance hormone levels.

Tears are the fluid of the Liver. We have a tendency in our society to view crying as a sign of sadness, and certainly there is a correlation in acute situations. But what about the person who starts to cry for no apparent reason, or who is simply prone to depression? In these instances, it is important to apply Energetics. Because tears are the fluid of the Liver, inexplicable crying or crying disproportionately related to a situation is a sign that the Liver is not performing optimally. Similarly, bouts of depression indicate that a Liver is not performing well. Your body attempts to dissipate emotional charge—often frustration, anger, and mood instability—with tears.

As final reminders, the health of the Liver can be viewed in the whites of the eyes, also known as the sclera. A red presentation reveals damage in the Liver, while a yellow presentation reveals jaundice and Liver congestion, which typically manifests as blocked Bile Ducts. The health of the Wood Element also can be viewed in the health of Tendons and Ligaments. Anyone with frequent muscle pulls, sprained ankles, or torn Ligaments—especially resulting from minimal physical stress at the time of injury—is revealing a congested Liver and blocked Bile Ducts associated and the Gallbladder.

Energetics: Wood Element Example

Your sister is thirty-two years old, and she had to have her Gallbladder removed about three years ago due to an accumulation of gallstones. A longtime sufferer of PMS symptoms, she often experiences bloating, mood instability, and breast tenderness. In her college years, she played basketball for two years until repeated ankle sprains and a torn ACL forced her to end her playing days. Most days she seems patient—until about five days before her period. During those five days, she's not much fun to be around. The last time you saw her, you noticed her eyes were really red from seasonal allergies.

Which Organs Are Involved?

1. Gallbladder Removal. **Liver, Gallbladder, Reproductive Glands**

2. Mood Instability. **Liver, Gallbladder, Reproductive Glands**

3. Bloating. **Acute Overgrowth of Intestinal Bacteria and Water Retention**

4. Breast Tenderness. **Acidic Cellular Environments**

5. Sprains and ACL Tears. **Liver, Gallbladder, Reproductive Glands**

6. Ankle Injury. **Kidney**

7. Red Eyes and Seasonal Allergies. **Liver, Gallbladder, Reproductive Glands**

Energetics: Accessory Fire Element

Yin Organ	Pericardium
Yang Organ	Triple Heater- Hypothalamus Pituitary Axis (HPAxis)
Gland	Hypothalamus Pituitary Axis (HPAxis)
Energetic Associations	Iris of Eyes (where the color is), Body Temperature
Fluids	Cerebrospinal Fluid
Tissues	Dura Mater, Glands
Time	Pericardium 7 P.M. – 9 P.M., Triple Heater 9 P.M. – 11 P.M.
Flavor	N/A
Energy-Draining Reactions	Alone, Isolated, Neglected, Guilty, Excessive Thought
Energy-Cultivating Responses	Investing Time In Life Passions, Family, and Friends

What's Interesting?

What I've often found intriguing about this element is its association with the Fire Element, and therefore, the Heart and Small Intestines. In your body, so many things are connected in a variety of ways, and some with a redundancy that overlaps other existing connections. I can only surmise that these redundancies exist in the event that something malfunctions. If a redundancy occurs in the physical body, then it would only make sense for it to occur in the energetic body as well. With a redundancy, life can continue.

What I've also found interesting is the relationship between the pericardium and the dural tissue. While the dural tissue envelops the Brain and a portion of the Spinal Cord, the pericardium envelops the Heart. Both create a sac-like enclosure that allows fluid to nourish, buffer, and protect the organs within. And both tissues—pericardium and dural tissue—have innervated collagen fibers that allow for contraction of the tissue. When a person experiences heartbreak, the pericardium actually begins to twist as it contracts as a means of protection. Similarly, the dural tissue contracts during heartbreak, and as it twists, it creates a phenomenon referred to as dural torque. Both tissues need to be able to contract, because under normal daily functioning, their ability to contract helps distribute blood and fluids to the contents they protect. However, when a person experiences heartbreak, the amount of torque generated by the adverse experience is enough for a person to experience chest-clutching pain or severe headaches.

This is another example of how emotion can turn into physical reality.

Life Lessons for Energy Cultivation

The Accessory Fire Element teaches us the importance of connection in everything we do. The Triple Heater-HPAxis is the gland that orchestrates virtually all hormonal functioning in the body, and as a result, fosters connectedness within the body. Similarly, when you spend time investing in your dreams, family, friends, and community, you are nurturing connections. When we are connected, we feel good, and we feel like there is a great deal to look forward to. Connection helps us maintain our enthusiasm, and this engages Energy-Cultivating Responses that support the actual Fire Element. As we will discuss in Volume 3, what we often refer to as networking helps create the opportunity for Win-Win-Win scenarios to appear—a win for you, a win for the other parties directly involved, and a win for everyone affected by your mutual agreement. When we are connected, opportunities are created that allow you to experience life. Everyone should be able to fully experience life for all its limitless possibilities.

And When Things Go Wrong

There are several situations and emotions that can lead to an imbalance in this particular element, including feeling lonely, isolated, guilty or neglected. These may be the most common, but first, let's discuss the difference between excessive concentration (Earth Element) and excessive thought (Accessory Fire Element). Excessive thought creates Cycles of Redundancy whereby a person replays negative experiences over and over and over and over, trying to achieve some semblance of satisfaction.

Let me give you an example of a situation we have all found ourselves in at one time or another. One fine afternoon you are humming along in your own world, when you suddenly encounter a person who catches you off guard and says something offensive. Now, perhaps they didn't even realize they were offending you, but it still bothered you. Dumbfounded, you stand there as the offending person trots away. And as you stand there, your emotions begin to get the best of you, and you start to realize that you just stood there and took it—that you didn't even say anything back. Now you're frustrated at the situation and disappointed in yourself for not jumping to your own defense.

The day goes on, work is over, and you get into your car. You suddenly notice that of all the cars in the parking lot, a pigeon decided to target your window. As you drive off in your private meditation chamber on wheels, what do you start doing? You start replaying the event that disrupted your day, right? You start replaying what that person said to you, and then you start thinking about what you *should* have said in response. You think to yourself, *Oh, if I would have said this, oh that would have been such a good comeback*. And a smile comes over your face. You have just discharged some emotion, but then you realize that you didn't actually say what you should have said to the person, so your replay and clever mental retort is unsatisfying. It is as unsatisfying as eating rice cakes when you're really starving for steak.

So what do you do? You have all this energy built up inside, and a great retort that you didn't use when you had the opportunity. You have been wronged and you are offended. Now you have this great comeback, but the moment when you could have used it passed hours ago. You can't call the person who offended you, so it's not possible to get your satisfaction that way. So what do you do? Thank God for cell phones, because talking to yourself in your vehicle makes people driving next to you a little nervous. You call up a friend—or whoever you talk to when you need to let off some steam—and you tell them the story. "Guess what happened to me today?"

Now here's where it gets funny. I love this part. You tell them the story, but now with a little twist. Embellishment time. You tell a little white lie, including what you should have said. Sometimes you tell your listener that you didn't actually use the comeback, but sometimes you make it seem like you actually said it. Why do you do the latter? So you can attempt to experience a little satisfaction. Then your listener says something like, "Ohhh, you thought of that? That was an awesome comeback." And you agree, but you have a little secret and you're still not feeling satisfied. So what do you do? You start thinking about the situation all over again. You have created a Cycle of Redundancy (See **Figure 6.2**), thanks to the excessive mental replay and your inability to forgive yourself for not having the witty comeback at the ready hours earlier.

This is precisely what excessive thought is—the search for satisfaction through mental replays. *Whenever you create a Cycle of Redundancy, you have engaged excessive thought in an attempt to create the satisfaction necessary to free up your energy for other things. Until you achieve satisfaction, the Cycle of Redundancy will remain.* This differs from excessive concentration, because excessive concentration pertains to prolonged periods of mental focus, whereas excessive thought pertains to mental replay in the pursuit of satisfaction.

Figure 6.2

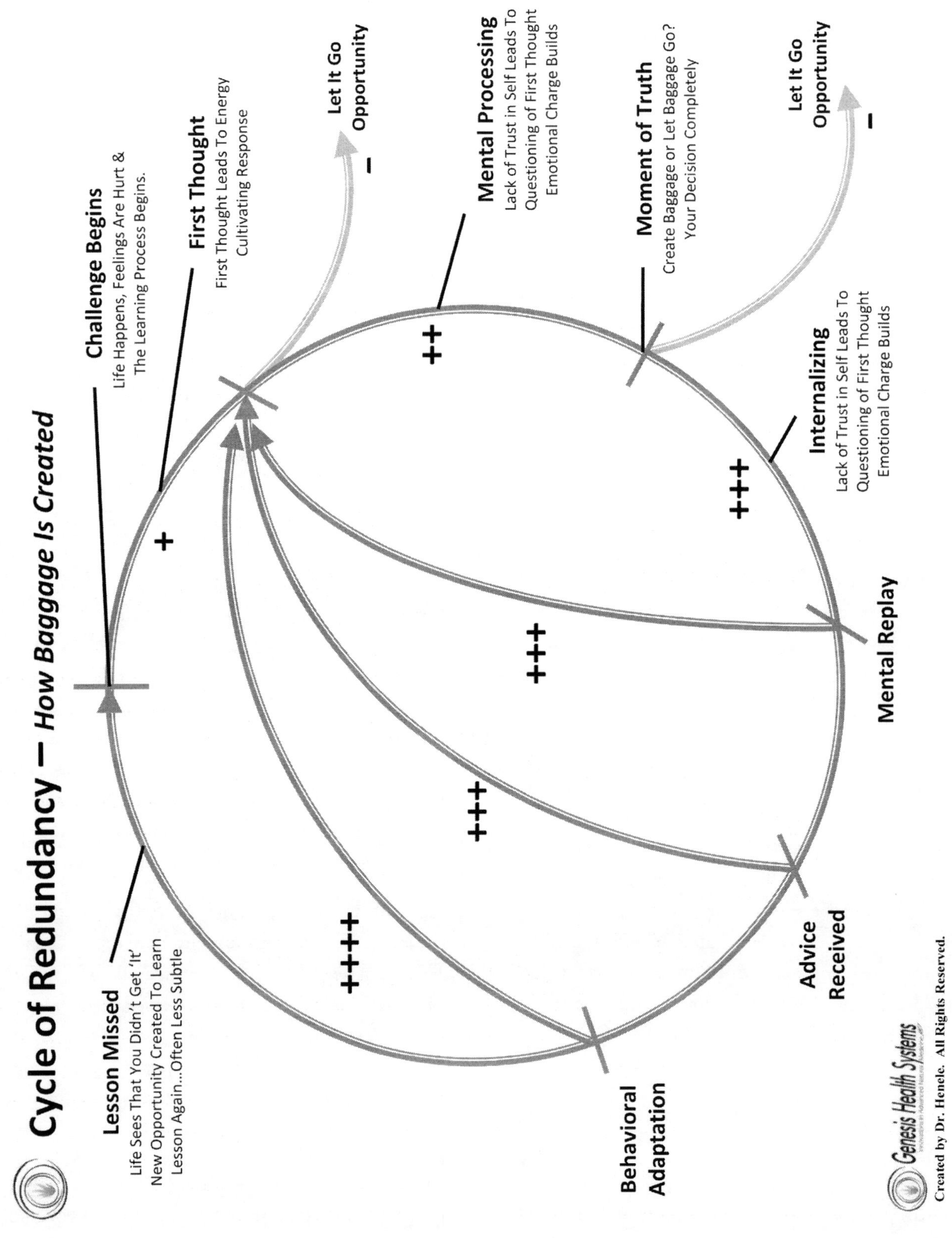
Cycle of Redundancy — How Baggage Is Created
Challenge Begins
Life Happens, Feelings Are Hurt & The Learning Process Begins.
First Thought
First Thought Leads To Energy Cultivating Response
Let It Go Opportunity
Mental Processing
Lack of Trust in Self Leads To Questioning of First Thought Emotional Charge Builds
Moment of Truth
Create Baggage or Let Baggage Go? Your Decision Completely
Let It Go Opportunity
Internalizing
Lack of Trust in Self Leads To Questioning of First Thought Emotional Charge Builds
Mental Replay
Advice Received
Behavioral Adaptation
Lesson Missed
Life Sees That You Didn't Get 'It' New Opportunity Created To Learn Lesson Again...Often Less Subtle
Genesis Health Systems
Created by Dr. Henele. All Rights Reserved.

Additional Associations

The Accessory Fire Element does not have a taste associated with it, so one could assume safely that the bitter flavor from the Fire Element also would stimulate this accessory element. Similarly, the time at which this element peaks in its energetic output is not important.

However, there are two associations that are of interest. The first is the association of the Iris. When we reviewed the Wood Element, we noted that the whites of the eyes revealed the health of the Liver. When assessing the Accessory Fire Element, make note that the Iris reveals the health of the Hypothalamus-Pituitary Axis. When the eyes are cloudy, this sign demonstrates a body that has been Bio-accumulating environmental pollution for quite some time. In the practice of Iridology, cloudy eyes are known as a lymphatic rosary, and they show when the Lymphatic chain is congested. What is it congested with? Environmental pollution. Where does this show up? In the Iris of the eye.

The second association that is of interest is body temperature. Body temperature is regulated by Thyroid Hormone. What's interesting about this is that it is the Pituitary Gland that signals the Thyroid Gland to release or not to release Thyroid Hormone. Thus, the true regulation of body temperature comes from the Hypothalamus-Pituitary Axis.

Energetics: Accessory Fire Element Example

For some strange reason, its Friday night and you find yourself at a supermarket around 11 P.M. Let's say it's a diaper run. Standing in front of you in the checkout line is an elderly woman who has a few Skin tags, Liver spots, and a noticeable Dowager's Hump. She is putting can after can of cat food on the conveyor belt, and then stops to see what you are doing. When you make eye contact, you notice that her eyes appear gray and cloudy. You smile, but she does not return the smile, choosing instead to resume putting her cat food on the conveyor belt. You notice that she doesn't even speak to the cashier who also attempts to greet her.

Which Organs Are Involved?

1. Skin Tags. **Insulin Resistance**
2. Liver Spots. **Liver, Gallbladder, Reproductive Glands**
3. Dowager's Hump (Kyphosis). **Lungs, Large Intestine, Thyroid, Parathyroid**
4. Gray, Cloudy Eyes. **Pericardium, Triple Heater-HPAxis**
5. Doesn't Return Smile or Greeting—Isolated. **Pericardium, Triple Heater-HPAxis**

Energy Pathway Meridians

Energy is the same thing as the *Vis Medicatrix Naturae*, also known as the *Vis*. The *Vis* is the same as the vital force, which is the same as *Chi* from Traditional Chinese Medicine, which is the same as *Prana* from Ayurvedic Medicine, which is the same as ATP from Western Biochemistry. Energy is energy is energy, regardless of what we call it.

So have you ever felt energy surge through your body? Perhaps you felt it when you were competing in sports, or before you gave a big performance. Maybe it happened while you were avoiding an auto accident. Or maybe it happened during one of those moments when you couldn't locate your toddler, and you were running around the house in a frenzied panic. And then you find your toddler banging on the hood of your new prized cherry inferno red Chrysler 300 with a hammer, and of course, with an innocent smile.

In Western society, science tries very hard to reduce this surge of *Chi* to an adrenaline rush. Is adrenaline rushing through your veins in an effort to stimulate Mitochondrial Energy Production? Absolutely. But there's much more going on than just adrenaline.

Throughout your body, there are definitive energy pathways that allow *Chi* to move through your body and reach every single cell. If you have more than 60,000 miles of blood vessels under your Skin, then why is it so hard to believe that energy pathways exist? If you've felt waves of heat or butterflies when in love, then why is it so difficult to believe in *Chi*? Because we can't see *Chi*? I can't see the future either, but I know it exists.

My point is this: Energy pathways—called meridians—exist whether science acknowledges them or not. Thankfully, most biochemists do acknowledge the existence of some force that orchestrates the countless number of reactions taking place within your body, every moment of every day. If you doubt the existence of energy pathway meridians, that's okay. Check out Bio Meridian Scanning (www.BioMeridian.com), because the technology actually exists today to prove the existence of meridians.

Now stepping off that little soapbox, let's talk about some AWESOME stuff. I want you to understand how *Chi* originates, how it flows into the meridian, and then how the meridians connect. This is important to understand, because it helps explain all of the energetic associations that make up the 5-Element Perspective.

Meridians form a three-dimensional blueprint for all physical development, growth, and healing. The prime example of this is Kirlian photography. Kirlian photography is a photography technique that allows you to take pictures of the energy fields that exist around all things. One of my favorite Kirlian photos is of a man who had his hand amputated. Sounds gruesome, but it's not. The Kirlian photograph revealed a pseudo-energetic hand even though the physical hand was no longer present. What this implies is that there exists a blueprint for our bodies, and it explains why humans usually have two arms, two legs, a torso, a head, and a neck. It helps explain why recent amputees can still feel the area where their amputated limb used to be. The suggestion is that we feel with much more than our Nervous Systems, and much more than our physical bodies.

Without the 3-D blueprint provided by the meridians of your body, your cells would not have the structure inside them to organize properly. As a result, we would undoubtedly look much different, and with a limitless amount of physical variation. It is the meridian that first forms the blueprint that attracts cells to specific locations during fetal development. The energy fields guide cells so they know which direction to grow in and how to transform. And we see this happening from the earliest moments of embryonic development and cellular transformation.

One of the most beautiful things that I ever studied in life was embryology. In every class, it was so much fun to watch this 3-D blueprint at work, preparing the physical body to receive the spiritual essence. With each day comes new and significant physical changes, and one can't help but wonder, *How in the heck does a cell know to go there? How does that cell know when to divide, and then do that, and then divide into this transformative thing? And how does it know to recreate this structure all the time? What is the inherent intelligence?* Well, the best thing I have ever been able to come up with is that the inherent intelligence comes from the energy pathways, referred to in the East as meridians.

From the time we are conceived, the energy fields go to work to create the necessary 3-D blueprint to help shape the human body. If the cellular environment is even close to ideal and the mother's and father's genetics are strong, then this process is designed to take place without error. However, if the mother's body is heavy with environmental pollution or infections, or if the father's genome is injured from the stress he has endured, then the possibility for error rises substantially.

When we look at a human body, what we are actually looking at is the densest form of energy. The physical body is the densest form of energy, but it is energy nonetheless As such, this brings us to the **Principle of Advanced Natural Medicine #28**: *The body is the densest form of energy, and as such, is the last place where degenerative disease will typically show itself. Degenerative disease can be traced back to its beginning, the disrupted flow of energy, and the Energy-Draining Reactions that result.*

Translated, this means that disease begins with fatigue, and the Energy-Draining Reactions that ensue. Disease begins on the energetic level, and when looking again at the Cycle of Influencing Energy®, Energetics influences emotion. Therefore, emotion becomes a perfect tool for assessment, particularly when lab tests show no abnormalities. It's no accident that you will feel problems forming in your physical body before they show up on lab reports. Your body is designed to work that way. In no way is this to diminish the importance of lab work, but to offer insight and an assurance that you are not crazy if you feel something going on, but a doctor can't find the problem. In many instances, you are perceiving the problem before it shows up in labwork. You are perceiving your energy fields.

This concept of perception becoming reality also supports the importance of awareness, and the control it offers over the expression of your emotional state. It is through the mastery of your emotions—by deciding to engage in Energy-Cultivating Responses as opposed to being a slave (and I am using that word on purpose), to Energy-Draining Reactions.

Understanding meridians and their 3-D blueprint, there are two primary meridian energy pathways to make note of—the internal meridians and the surface meridians. The flow of energy through meridians begins within the organ for which the meridian is named. As Mitochondria produce energy in the form of ATP, the energy signature of the ATP that forms is referred to as *Chi*. *Chi* collects within the cells of an organ, and then it enters the internal meridian for that organ, which extends from the organ to its surface meridian. Energy from the internal meridian enters the surface meridian at what is known as a source point. It is from the study of meridian *Chi* flow that Acupuncture is built on, and why an acupuncturist will work to stimulate your digestion by inserting a needle into your arm or leg. What they are doing is stimulating the energy pathway associated with the sick organ. Again, when you assess health, first figure out which organ or organs are affected, as this is the key to developing treatment strategies.

The organ and the cells contained within it are where all the magic begins. Organs with healthy Mitochondrial populations, low stress, and an abundance of nutrients will have more energy, filling both the internal meridian and the surface meridian. *If the organ is strong, the meridian is going to be strong. If the organ is weak and diseased, then the meridian will be weak and diseased.* Every meridian associated with an organ has a source point where energy enters the channel from the internal meridian. Meridians are bilateral, meaning that for each organ, there is a meridian on each side of the body designed to create balance.

Looking at the source points in a little more detail, source points are placed on the body and help assess the health of the underlying organ. If the source point for an organ's meridian is soft, or feels like a divot, then the body is revealing an organ that is deficient in energy production. Conversely, if a source point for an organ's meridian is hard or stiff, this reveals an organ that is imbalanced and in excess, meaning this organ is compensating for a deficiency elsewhere in the body. Without getting to heavy into the philosophy of Traditional Chinese Medicine, know that your body seeks balance, regardless of whether we are talking about the Anatomy of posture, the Biochemistry of ATP production, or Energetics. Any imbalance on any level forces your body to compensate, and that leads to more imbalances. The role of the healer is to find the imbalances (obstacles to cure) and remove them. When imbalances are removed and energy is present, health tends to be the result.

So please allow me to repeat myself and build on some earlier concepts. Organs cultivate energy at the Mitochondrial level. Energy signatures of ATP are collected within each organ, and they enter the internal meridian as *Chi*. *Chi* flows through the internal meridian to the surface meridian, entering the surface meridian at the meridian's source point. And meridians are bilateral to create balance.

Surface meridians also are connected to each other in a specific pattern so that surface meridians receive *Chi* from the corresponding organ, and from the surface meridian that precedes them. Ultimately, we can look at this phenomenon in terms of circuits. There are three major energy circuits created by surface meridian connections (See **Figure 6.3**).

First Circuit

- Lung Meridians connect to Large Intestine Meridians
- Large Intestine Meridians connect to Stomach Meridians
- Stomach Meridians connect to Spleen-Pancreas Meridians
- Spleen-Pancreas Meridians connect to Heart Meridians

Second Circuit

- Heart Meridians connect to Small Intestine Meridians
- Small Intestine Meridians connect to Urinary Bladder Meridians
- Urinary Bladder Meridians connect to Kidney Meridians
- Kidney Meridians connect to Pericardium Meridians

Third Circuit

- Pericardium Meridians connect to Triple Heater-HPAxis Meridians
- Triple Heater-HPAxis Meridians connect to Gallbladder Meridians
- Gallbladder Meridians connect to Liver Meridians
- Liver Meridians connect back to Lung Meridians

What's wonderful about these surface connections is that they go full circle, and they allow every organ and Energetic to work in concert. There also are two additional channels called the Governing Vessel and the Conception Vessel that regulate energy flow through all of the meridians. These are most closely associated with the Rest-and-Digest Nervous System.

So what does all of this Energetics stuff mean to you? It means that wherever injuries or diseased tissues appear in the body, the injury or diseased tissue reveals exactly which organ or organs are involved, and as a result, which ones are in need of support. It is no accident that acne shows up on the face, rather than on the back of the knees. In the face are surface meridians for the organs associated with digestion, while along the back of the knee, are surface meridians for the Kidney and Urinary Bladder. Knowing how your body is designed three-dimensionally helps you make intelligent decisions. Before you understood how your body communicates with you, a Skin condition might have been just something on your Skin. Now that you have some knowledge and understanding about the fact that there are no accidents in the body, you now know that a problem with your Skin is revealing something that is going on deeper within your body. Now you can pinpoint the affected organ with the knowledge of where the corresponding meridian exists.

Final Thoughts on the Mastery of Emotion

Emotion is really a major foundation for the entire health of your body. You have a choice, you always have a choice. You can choose to master your emotions and be in control of them at all times, or you can choose to be a slave to them and risk feeling overwhelmed with the Energy-Draining Reactions.

If you choose to master emotions and utilize Energy-Cultivating Responses, does that mean that you are never going to get frustrated? Of course not! But it does mean that you don't have to be a slave to frustration, or allow your day to be ruined by it.

Certainly you must consider authenticity to make sure that whatever you are expressing is genuine. But the more you train yourself and develop this skill of Positive Internal Dialogue, the better you will become at utilizing Change It as a reflex, and the more you will be able to master your life and generate Energy-Cultivating Responses as a habit.

Figure 6.3

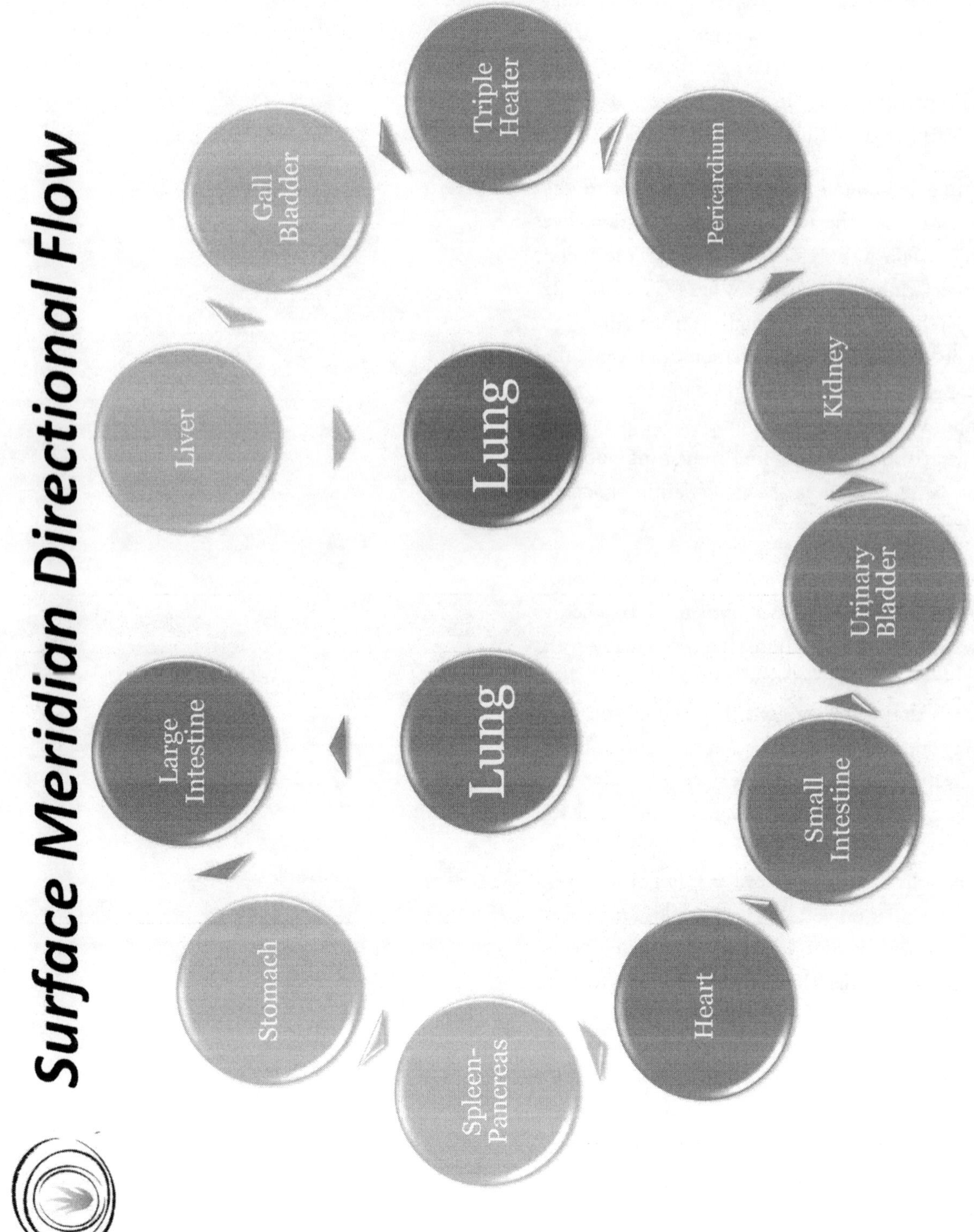
Surface Meridian Directional Flow
Lung
Large Intestine
Stomach
Spleen-Pancreas
Heart
Small Intestine
Urinary Bladder
Kidney
Pericardium
Triple Heater
Gall Bladder
Liver
Lung

The foundation—the building block for all of Advanced Natural Medicine—starts with finding something good in all things regardless of the situation. It doesn't matter what you are presented with, what matters is that you find something good as a habit. All good things come to those who earn them, and when you find something good in your life every day, you are truly earning good things.

Healing is about earning your health, and the journey within. All the answers to your questions live inside you. Make a conscious effort each day to spend time appreciating and enjoying What's Good in your life—everything from the people you encounter to the silly little things. This appreciation can include the apple that you just ate, and things we too often ignore like simply waking up. The triumphs, the pain—no matter what the situation—find something good in them all, because there is always something good to be discovered.

On some level, we are all children of a Higher Power—a Higher Power that radiates love energy in every conceivable direction. The love energy feels so good, it only hurts when we think it's gone. But the truth is that it's never gone. Every time you find something good, you connect back to the source of love energy. Every time you appreciate something silly, you reconnect with your Higher Power and the father we all share. And when you're still enough, quiet enough, happy enough, this force of love energy talks to you, guides you, smiles on you. In these precious moments you are connected, and you are experiencing what mastery of life means. The only difference between a master and one who has yet to master is the ability to reconnect within the span of a single breath. That's it. In this way, a master is imminently predictable. The master is not attracted to life as a slave, as one who does not believe or feel worthy enough to make the connection. The master makes the same decision every time, because the decision is rewarded with the experience of love energy.

Listening to Your Amazing Body

As we come to a close with the Volume 1, understand that everything your body says provides useful information when you learn its language and know how to interpret it. Fatigue, the Cycle of Influencing Energy®, the 4 Considerations for Healing, Mitochondrial Energy Production, Eating Healthy, and Energetics all teach you the language that you need to interpret what your body is telling you. Understanding the body's language and what it is saying to you will help you make excellent, knowledgeable decisions regarding your health. As good decisions accumulate, so does the momentum you will need to realize your dreams in this lifetime.

FIRE ELEMENT

A 'Yes' answer to any of the following questions suggests an imbalance in the Fire Element.

1. Have you recently been through a breakup or lost a loved one?

   Yes No

2. Do you believe yourself to be unworthy of love?

   Yes No

3. Do you have a difficult time with change?

   Yes No

4. Would you say that you are quick to give up?

   Yes No

5. Does your tongue have a large crack down the middle?

   Yes No

6. Do you notice your voice cracking?

   Yes No

7. Are you frequently asked to speak louder?

   Yes No

8. Do you sweat less than three times per week?

   Yes No

9. Have you ever been diagnosed with a Heart ailment?

   Yes No

EARTH ELEMENT

A 'Yes' answer to any of the following questions suggests an imbalance in the Earth Element.

1. Do you concentrate for more than six hours per workday?

   Yes No

2. Are you easily overwhelmed?

   Yes No

3. Do you purposely stay busy?

   Yes No

4. Does it take you longer than fifteen minutes to get to sleep at night?

   Yes No

5. Do you have any regular digestive issues?

   Yes No

6. Do you bruise easily?

   Yes No

7. Do you regularly have loose stools?

   Yes No

8. Do you have heartburn or take antacids?

   Yes No

9. Do you crave sweets or soda frequently throughout your day?

   Yes No

GOLD ELEMENT

A 'Yes' answer to any of the following questions suggests an imbalance in the Gold Element.

1. Do you have a history of Asthma or respiratory disease?

   Yes No

2. Do you have a history of colitis or constipation?

   Yes No

3. Would you describe yourself as 'pleasing'?

   Yes No

4. Do you refrain from speaking your mind out of consideration for others?

   Yes No

5. Do you have a difficult time letting go of bad experiences?

   Yes No

6. Do you frequently get sick?

   Yes No

7. Do you frequently wake up between 3 A.M. and 5 A.M.?

   Yes No

8. Do you crave hot and spicy foods?

   Yes No

9. Do you frequently talk to yourself in a negative way?

   Yes No

WATER ELEMENT

A 'Yes' answer to any of the following questions suggests an imbalance in the Water Element.

1. Do you frequently develop urinary tract infections?

   Yes No

2. Does it take one or more cups of coffee to get going in the morning?

   Yes No

3. Would you describe yourself as fearful?

   Yes No

4. Would you describe yourself as anxious?

   Yes No

5. Do you have to have everything exactly your way to be happy?

   Yes No

6. Do you hear a ringing in your ears regularly?

   Yes No

7. Has your libido diminished noticeably?

   Yes No

8. Any history of bone cancer or frequently broken bones?

   Yes No

9. Do you crave salty foods?

   Yes No

WOOD ELEMENT

A 'Yes' answer to any of the following questions suggests an imbalance in the Wood Element.

1. Is it difficult to place you fingers underneath your rib cage?

   Yes No

2. Have you had your Gallbladder removed or been diagnosed with gallstones?

   Yes No

3. Are you easily frustrated?

   Yes No

4. Do you get impatient in traffic or with slow drivers?

   Yes No

5. Do you find yourself complaining frequently?

   Yes No

6. Do you have PMS, mood instability, or heavy periods?

   Yes No

7. Have you ever torn a Tendon or Ligament?

   Yes No

8. Do you frequently wake up between 1 A.M. and 3 A.M.?

   Yes No

9. Does it take you awhile to decide on a meal?

   Yes No

ACCESSORY FIRE ELEMENT

A 'Yes' answer to any of the following questions suggests an imbalance in the Accessory Fire Element.

1. Any history of smoking?

   Yes No

2. Any history of Brain tumors?

   Yes No

3. Do you feel alone, neglected, or guilty?

   Yes No

4. Do you find yourself replaying the day's events frequently?

   Yes No

5. Do you avoid going out with friends and family?

   Yes No

6. Are your eyes cloudy?

   Yes No

What You Can Do To Cultivate Energy Today

Practicing Change It with Pre-Programming. Pre-Programming is a technique for understanding where you are frequently losing energy, and deciding how you are going to Change It beforehand so that you are prepared for success. We have been secretly doing a little of this with each new resolution, but let's roll the whole thing out now.

Change It with Pre-Programming

1. Identify where you are losing energy by identifying your stressor before you are in the challenging situation.
2. Breathe until you know exactly how you want to respond to the stress.
3. Practice Positive Internal Dialogue and encourage yourself.
4. Give yourself a Mental High Five.
5. In the moment, breathe and draw on your Pre-Programmed Response. Trust it, believe in it, and use it.
6. Practice Positive Internal Dialogue and encourage yourself.
7. Give yourself another Mental High Five. You can't give yourself enough Mental High-Fives in a day—they're like antioxidants for your mind.

RESOLUTION #9

Select two Stressors and Pre-Program your response to them. At the same time, be sure to give yourself as many Mental High-Fives as you need to build and retain your confidence.

Stressor #1

1. ______________________________

Pre-Programmed Response

2. ______________________________

Stressor #2

1. ______________________________

Pre-Programmed Response

2. ______________________________

HEALING JOURNAL RECORDING

Record in your Healing Journal your moods, thoughts, and positive experiences throughout the week. Pay special attention to how well you are developing your Change It skill, and what you are feeling about some of the things you read in this chapter. Keep developing your ability to spend more time discovering What's Good.

Good Luck!

ALKALIZING HEALING PLAN

	Therapy	Instructions
Primary Therapy	Organic Clinical Nutrition	Continue Eating Healthy.
Complementary Therapy	Breathing Practice	Upon waking and before starting your morning routine, breathe for thirty to forty-five minutes, listening to your breath while inhaling and exhaling. Get stronger.
Complementary Therapy	Yoga	Activate your feet frequently throughout the day while standing, walking, or sitting.
Complementary Therapy	Exercise	Exercise using the method or variety of methods of your choice. The goal is a minimum of thirty minutes from the time you begin to perspire, three to five times this week.
Essential Therapy	Sleep	Commit to a minimum of seven hours of sleep each night, and give yourself one day each week to sleep until your body is ready to wake up.
Essential Therapy	Positive Internal Dialogue	Work on your skill to Change It. Give yourself an abundance of Mental High-Fives.

VOLUME 1 COMPLEMENTARY INFORMATION

Nutrient-Dosing Strategies, Definitions, and Summary of Healing Principles

Interesting Insights to look for in this section:

- Why underdosing makes natural medicine look bad.
- Innovative dosing strategies.
- What's a hiccup?
- Summary of Principles of Advanced Natural Medicine.

Principle of Advanced Natural Medicine #29:

The single most important factor in healing plan development is achieving Therapeutic Range for Mitochondrial Energy Production.

Underdosing—The Most Common Error in Natural Medicine

It's not enough to simply take a certain nutrient or herb. We have to take nutrients and herbs properly at the right times, and at the right dosages needed to achieve a Therapeutic Range. When discussing underdosing, there are a couple of things that are important to understand.

The first is that we live in a quick-fix society. As a result, we don't often give our bodies enough time to figure out what to do with new nutrients and healing plans. It's expected that as soon as something is swallowed...PRESTO! We should be all better. Well, your body just doesn't work that way. Recall that your body is designed to heal in twenty-eight-day cycles. As such, twenty-eight days is the minimum amount of time before a professional or anyone can accurately assess the effectiveness of a particular treatment. If something good happens before the twenty-eight days is up, fantastic! It's a win, so take it.

But if the gains are small within the first two weeks, this could simply be because your cells are trying to figure out how to use what you've started giving them. Remember, the process of producing energy is dependent on a bunch of enzymes within the cell that accelerate biochemical reactions. Well, what if your body hasn't been producing those enzymes consistently for the past couple of years, and now you're making some changes? You'll need to give your body more than two weeks to figure out how to make that an efficient process again. I hope that makes some sense. After twenty-eight days you can adequately assess the progress and ask: "Did the changes made have a positive effect?" Making assessments before the end of the twenty-eight-day period would be premature.

Underdosing Error #1. All the essential nutrients for Mitochondrial Energy Production are not dosed, or if they are—which so seldom happens—other key nutrients or botanical medicines are missing. Marketing is great when it comes to creating the next GREATEST THING EVER. Years ago, it was aloe vera juice, then noni juice, then mangostein, then resveratrol, then Quercetin. Can you see the problem with this? The marketing agencies are creating hype, and as a result, setting people up for a big letdown. But why should they care? They were in it for the money. Now a person has a big bottle of something with a recommended dose that is ineffective. Why? Because they don't have the nutrients essential for their Mitochondria, and the product isn't even in the Therapeutic Range for optimal dosing. As a result, people conclude it doesn't work. Of course it doesn't work—the situation had failure written all over it!

But what if you were taking the GREATEST THING EVER at the correct dose, and with all the nutrients you needed for optimal energy production? Think your opinion might be a little different?

Underdosing Error #2. The correct nutrients are selected but not taken in a dose high enough to enter into the Therapeutic Range. Let's say, for example, that someone has bleeding gums and they correctly select Vitamin C as a target nutrient. Let's also say that they are taking everything their Mitochondria need to produce energy. The Therapeutic Range for Vitamin C is 2,000 to 4,000 milligrams per day taken in divided doses. But this person is taking only 500 milligrams per day. They did 90 percent of everything right, but dropped the ball on making sure they achieved Therapeutic Range. And the end result is their conclusion: "This natural medicine stuff doesn't work."

How could this be? Doesn't every single supplement company know about the Therapeutic Range? Aren't all of the dosing recommendations established for Therapeutic Range? Hardly. Most companies copy other companies, leaving the consumer high and dry. What most of them—but not all of them—are concerned with is getting you to use the supplement bottle in one month's time so that you will buy another bottle.

What's worse is that most supplement companies make products for mass consumption, and are not concerned about the quality of their product or the absorption rates. Sadly, most of the products available for mass consumption are high-priced junk.

Underdosing Error #3. Nutrients are not dosed frequently enough to sustain healing resonance. So let's say that a person has selected the right nutrients for their Mitochondria and for their target specific condition. And let's also say they've even had nutrients in the correct Therapeutic Range. The next big error is that most people don't dose themselves with enough frequency to maintain adequate levels of these nutrients in their bloodstream.

Now, natural or not, your body is always working to achieve a balance—particularly in your bloodstream. When you take a cluster of nutrients, for example, they are hopefully absorbed at a high rate and carried through the bloodstream to the targeted cells. Over the course of several hours, the bloodstream is constantly filtered by the Liver and Kidneys to maintain a healthy alkaline pH of 7.35 to 7.45. As your cells use the nutrients, and as your Liver and Kidneys filter the blood, the amount of nutrients available for your cells will dwindle in the hours after your last dosing. So it stands to reason that there's a strong likelihood that what you dosed at 8 a.m. is not substantially available for your cells by 8 P.M. Falling victim to this underdosing error also can lead a person to think: *This natural stuff doesn't work.*

Underdosing Error #4. Premature termination of the healing nutrients or the healing plan. A person who doesn't feel the benefit of the changes they are making is more likely to discontinue the changes, particularly if money becomes an issue. The responsibility of every person—whether that person is the physician or the patient—is to have a clear outline of expectations. If a person expected that natural medicine was going to produce instant and lasting results in a single day, then good luck on that one. Healing takes time. Give change at least twenty-eight days before you decide whether it has been effective or not.

I've heard too many people say things like the following before they start working with me: "I tried this stuff and it didn't work. I tried to exercise and I felt worse. I tried this supplement and I felt worse. I tried this supplement and I didn't feel anything. I tried changing my diet and I didn't feel anything, I didn't lose any weight."

My response to them is always: "Did you give it enough time? How long did you try it for?" What I hear most of the time is, "Well, I tried it for seven days, ten days." Okay, hmmmm, that's good, I guess. Then I teach them what their body needs and why.

Because it's one thing to realize a positive benefit; it's an entirely different thing for your body to maintain it. Remember that we are basing the foundation of health on energy production. The goal is to make sure that an effect is felt within the first twenty-eight days—and really within the first two weeks, if the situation allows you to dose with some vigor. My goal with every patient is to have them feel a positive effect within two weeks, and certainly within twenty-eight days. I'd rather have my patients feel something early in the first twenty-eight day healing cycle than risk my patient feeling nothing. Let me say that again. When I dose my patients—especially when they're starting their initial healing program—I give them a lot. I dose them up. And I dose them up, so that they feel something. I want them to feel a change in their health, because I know that if I can get somebody to feel something within two weeks, there's a strong likelihood that they're going to see the healing plan through to the healing resolution.

And after the healing resolution is achieved, the shift into maintenance dosing is a welcome reward for a job well done.

Therapeutic Range

Therapeutic Range is the amount of a nutrient required over the course of a day to ensure that healing resonance is achieved. The dosing recommended to enter Therapeutic Range is based on a typical 150-pound adult, but it also can be applied to a person who weighs between 125 and 200 pounds.

Nutrient	Single Nutrient Therapeutic Range
Vitamin B1, Thiamine	20—100 mg
Vitamin B2, Riboflavin	15—75 mg
Vitamin B3, Niacin	100—200 mg
Vitamin B5, Pantothenic Acid	100—400 mg
Vitamin B6, Pyridoxine	25—50 mg
Vitamin B12, Cobalamin	1,000—1,500 mcg
Folic Acid	800-2000 mcg
Biotin	200-800 mcg
Vitamin A, Retinol	10,000 IU
Vitamin A, Beta Carotene	Minimum 25,000 IU
Vitamin C, Ascorbic Acid	3,000-5,000 mg or higher
Vitamin D3	400—1,000 IU
Vitamin E	400—600 IU
Vitamin K	400—800 mcg
Magnesium	700—1,100 mg
Calcium	1,000—2,000 mg
Phosphorus	700—1,500 mg
Potassium	Minimum 4,700 mg
Sodium	3,800 mg
Iron	10—35 mg
Copper	0.7 to 2.5 mg
Zinc	11—40 mg
Selenium	75—200 mcg
Manganese	2—6 mg
Chromium	35—200 mcg
Molybdenum	35—200 mcg
Vanadium	20—100 mcg
Iodine	150—400 mcg
Silica	20—200 mg
Boron	2—4 mg
Inositol	1,000—2,000 mg
Choline	1,000—2,000 mg
Co-Q-10	100—300 mg
Alpha Lipoic Acid	400—1,200 mg
D-Ribose	10,000 mg or more
Quercetin	2,000—10,000 mg
Chlorophyll	2,000—6,000 mg
Resveratrol	100—300 mg
L-Carnitine	500—4,000 mg
N-Acetyl Cysteine	600—1,200 mg
L-Tryptophan	500—2,000 mg

Nutrient	Single Nutrient Therapeutic Range
L-Tyrosine	2,000—6,000 mg
L-Taurine	2,000—4,000 mg
L-Lysine	500—4,000 mg
L-Glutamine	3,000—4,000 mg
L-Methionine	3,000—6,000 mg
L-Proline	3,000—4,000 mg
EPA (Fish Oil)	400—800 mg
DHA (Fish Oil)	300—600 mg
Lactobacillus acidophilus	3 billion CFU or more
Lactobacillus casei	2 billion CFU or more
Bifidobacterium all	1 to 5 billion CFU or more
Phytonutrient Antioxidants	5—10 grams or more

Target Specific Nutrients and Herbs

Target specific nutrients and herbs have an affinity for certain organs and tissues, and they can help provide that little extra boost to the targeted area—provided that the Mitochondria receive everything they need to produce energy. Below is a small list of nutrients and herbs that fit this bill. If any doubt exists in their clinical application, please work with a licensed Naturopathic Physician and be sure that your Mitochondria have everything they need.

Target System	Nutrients and Herbs
Myofascial	Water, Vitamin C, Vitamin A, Quercetin, Silica, Proline, Omega 3 Fatty Acids, Zinc, Vitamin D, Calcium, Magnesium, Potassium, Sodium, Vitamin K, Burdock Root, Calendula
Nervous	Potassium, Sodium, Choline, Inositol, Essential Fatty Acids, Lecithin, Pantothenic Acid, Magnesium, Amino Acids, Quercetin, Skullcap, Rosemary, Passion Flower, Kava Kava
Immune	D-Beta Glucans, Vitamin A, Vitamin D, Vitamin C, Zinc, Reishi, Maitake, Shitake, Cordyceps, Astragalus Root, Allicin, Lauracidin, Licorice Root, Chlorophyll, Green Tea
Cardiovascular	Chlorophyll, Co-Q-10, Taurine, L-Carnitine, Essential Fatty Acids, Magnesium, Potassium, Vitamin E, Hawthorn Berry, Lemon Balm, Rosemary, Nettle Leaf
Digestive	L-Glutamine, Probiotics, Digestive Enzymes, Vitamin C, Dandelion Root, Milk Thistle, Lecithin, Essential Fatty Acids, Eating Healthy, Gentian Root, Peppermint, Spearmint
Respiratory	Vitamin A, Vitamin C, Zinc, N-Acetyl Cysteine, Glutathione, Quercetin, Pyridoxine, Lobelia, Mullein, Eucalyptus, Elderberries
Urinary	Water, Vitamin C, Potassium, Sodium, Biotin, Uva Ursi, Corn Silk
Hormonal	Trace Minerals, Amino Acids

Optimal Dosing Strategies for Advanced Natural Medicine

I love to put my patients in the best possible situation for success. The thought process that best enables this is to seek out fatigue and start from there. I implore you to use the Cycle of Influencing Energy®, the 4 Considerations for Healing, the keys for Mitochondrial Energy Production, Eating Healthy, and Energetics in the assessment of the problem and design of your healing plan. When you have a rationale for why you are doing what you are doing, it makes it much easier to adjust your healing plan and continue on the path of success.

Successful Thought Process for Nutrient and Herb Dosing

1. Dose nutrients essential for Mitochondrial Energy Production in Therapeutic Range.
2. Dose target specific nutrients and botanical medicines in Therapeutic Range.
3. Select correct dosing strategy or strategies.
4. Follow diligently for twenty-eight days before you reassess.

Dosing with Food

With the exception of dosing glandulars and enzymes for chronic inflammatory conditions, all nutrients and herbs should be dosed with a small amount of alkalizing food that contains some fiber. Fiber will help slow the absorption process and limit temporary bouts of nausea associated with elevated nutrient dosing.

A.M. DOSING

Morning A.M. Dosing is best utilized for cultivating energy throughout the workday. Dosing can occur with breakfast or with lunch depending on when the energy boost is needed. If you are more fatigued in the morning, then dose in the morning. If you are more fatigued in the early afternoon, dose with lunch.

P.M. DOSING

P.M. dosing is typically associated with dinner. While A.M. dosing is to provide energy throughout the workday, P.M. dosing is to provide the Immune System and your systems of detoxification with all the nutrients they need to do their jobs. P.M. dosing is a perfect time to dose Mitochondrial Nutrients.

BEFORE-BED DOSING

Before-Bed Dosing is fifteen to thirty minutes before bed. While P.M. dosing helps nourish your Mitochondria before your Immune System becomes active, it also is the ideal time to dose targeted nutrients for the Immune System. Before-Bed Dosing is essential for acute colds, cleansing, and all chronic conditions.

MAINTENANCE DOSING

Maintenance Dosing is fairly simple. Select either one A.M. or P.M. Dosing—depending on your preference—and dose nutrients and herbs once a day three to five times per week.

CELLULAR-CLEANSING DOSING

Optimally twenty-eight days of continual dosing, including an A.M. and P.M. Dosing. Some cleansing regimens also will include a third dosing in addition to dosing bentonite clay and psyllium upon waking, in the middle of the day, and before bed.

CHRONIC-CONDITION DOSING

When dosing for chronic conditions, it is essential to understand that this is for the long haul and that everyone needs a break—even from being sick. The body also needs a day to balance itself out, and to work on its own without all the nutrients and herbs. Chronic Condition Dosing is literally five to six days per week, only with an A.M. and a P.M. Dosing. This will allow the Liver and the Kidneys to keep the blood very clean without overworking them.

ACUTE-CONDITION DOSING

In order to achieve adequate blood levels of nutrients and herbal remedies for acute conditions, dosing should begin in earnest every two to three waking hours for a minimum of two days in what is called a loading dose. The dosing should then be maintained in Therapeutic Range two to three times per day, and continue for two days after you feel that the acute condition has resolved. This type of dosing typically does not last longer than seven days.

PEAK ATHLETIC PERFORMANCE DOSING

For optimal training regimens, all dosing of nutrients—especially Mitochondrial nutrients—should begin in earnest within thirty minutes of completing the training regimen. If the training regimen is to commence early in the morning, make sure to practice P.M. Dosing the night before to pre-load your body. On the actual days of competition, nutrient dosing should begin sixty minutes before the start of the event, and should resume within thirty minutes after the competition has concluded.

PARASITE DOSING

Parasites can include bacteria, viruses, fungi, spores, nematodes, and others. These little buggers can be very persistent, due to their ability to create bio-films and burrow deep into your subacute tissues. Therefore, dosing needs to be aggressive for two weeks, including all anti-microbials known to kill the specific bugs you are targeting for annihilation. Dietary considerations should be made to avoid refined sugar during this time. A Parasite Dosing cycle works like this: Two weeks of consistent A.M. and P.M, Dosing treatment, followed by one week off of the anti-microbials, but not the energy producing nutrients. So, one cycle is three weeks long. Most Parasite Dosing will require two to three cycles to achieve full effectiveness.

BENTONITE-CLAY DOSING

When using bentonite clay in cellular cleanses or with Parasite Dosing regimens, it is important to understand that bentonite clay is a powerful adsorber, meaning that it grabs everything good, bad, and ugly. With this in mind, it is important to make sure that you take bentonite clay a minimum of ninety minutes from the time that food, nutrients, and herbs are ingested.

GLANDULAR DOSING

Glandulars will compete with nutrients for absorption. As such, they should be dosed a minimum of thirty minutes before any food is eaten.

DIETARY-ENZYME DOSING

Enzymes used to enhance the digestive process should be taken either five minutes before your meal or within five minutes of beginning your meal. Digestive enzymes can still be effective outside of the five-minute window, and have been effective when taken within thirty minutes after finishing your meal.

ANTI-INFLAMMATORY ENZYME DOSING

Enzymes used to modulate a chronic inflammatory condition should always be taken at least ninety minutes—preferably two hours—from eating to optimize their effect.

BI-PHASIC DOSING

Bi-Phasic Dosing is utilized primarily as a strategy for working with imbalances in the female reproductive cycle. The female reproductive cycle can be segmented by ovulation into two phases—the follicular phase, and the luteal phase. With a knowledge of when ovulation is occurring, a skilled physician can intelligently dose with precise nutrient and botanical medicines for each phase, and in doing so, create healing resonance with great speed.

CHEMOTHERAPY DOSING

When dosing for chemotherapy, knowledge of the half-life of the chemotherapeutic agent is essential. Most chemotherapeutic agents will demonstrate a maximum efficacy of five half-lives. While the chemotherapeutic agent is biologically active, nutrients that cultivate energy can actually accelerate the clearance of the agent, and as a result, reduce its efficacy. For at least two weeks prior to chemotherapy, the participant should be A.M. and P.M. Dosing all nutrients essential for Mitochondrial Energy Production. On the day before the chemotherapy is administered, dosing for Mitochondrial

Energy Production should discontinue if the supervising oncologist wishes it to be so. At this time, it is safe to begin dosing at high levels of antioxidants and complete amino acids at A.M. and P.M. intervals, and up to four times a day, to help sustain the body during chemotherapy. Immediately following the end of the fifth half-life cycle of the chemotherapeutic agent, A.M. and P.M. Dosing with *ALL* the nutrients essential for Mitochondrial Energy Production should begin in earnest, along with target specific nutrients for supporting the Liver and Kidneys, at the very least. The idea is to significantly rebuild the body in between chemotherapy rounds. Dosing in between chemotherapy rounds also can safely increase to three to four times a day.

Essential Healing Definitions

Healing Process—What one enters into when they begin making positive lifestyle changes.

Healing Response—Formerly called Healing Crisis or Healing Reaction, neither of which sound attractive. Healing responses are good things. Temporary events that may at first feel adverse or challenging, but that ultimately help to open blocked energy fields.

Healing Resonance—The synergistic blending of multiple natural therapies and/or multiple nutrients and botanical medicines, allowing for the use of minimal therapeutic intervention without compromising maximum therapeutic effect. When healing resonance is achieved, the patient will feel a noticeable surge in energy and the Healing Process naturally will accelerate.

Healing Plateau—Stage of healing whereby no further improvements will be realized until new positive lifestyle changes are initiated. A healing plateau demands modifications to the healing plan design.

Healing Resolution—Finalization of Healing Process whereby the body's tissues have restored and strengthened themselves back to or close to their pre-injury/pre-diseased state.

Interpretations of Pain Descriptions and Common Physical Sensations

For more information about these and additional sensations, refer to the specific chapter in Volume 2 associated with the Thought Processes listed below.

SENSATION	THOUGHT PROCESS
Sharp, Shooting, Stabbing Pain	Think—Nervous System
Numbness, Loss of Sensation or Function	Think—Nervous System
Swollen Ankles	Think—Cardiovascular System and Lymphatic, Immune System
Muscle Spasms	Think—Stagnant Lymphatic System
Hiccups	Think—Stagnant Lymphatic System and Atrophied Diaphragm
Dull, Achy, Migrating Pain	Think—Myofascial System and Adhesions (Scar Tissue)
Bloating	Think—Digestive System and Bacterial/Fungal Overgrowth
Smelly Poop	Think—It's Time for a Twenty-Eight-Day Cellular Cleanse
Farts that Smell	Think—Digestive System and Bacterial/Fungal Overgrowth
Mucus Anywhere	Think—Acidic Cellular Environments, Tissue Damage, Inflammation
Tender Skin, Red Skin	Think—Acidic Cellular Environments
Joint Pain	Think—Delayed Food Allergies

Principles of Advanced Natural Medicine

Principle of Advanced Natural Medicine #1:

Where there is space, there is movement.
Where there is movement, there is energy.
Where there is energy, disease cannot exist.

Principle of Advanced Natural Medicine #2:

Your body is designed to heal. Sophisticated Simplicity makes it all possible.

Principle of Advanced Natural Medicine #3:

First, treat the body from the inside out. Second, treat the body from the outside in. Third, participate and move.

Principle of Advanced Natural Medicine #4:

Your body does not differentiate between various types of stress. Stress from internalized emotion causes just as much cellular damage as stress from acidic diets. The body responds to all stresses in similar fashion—by garnering its energetic resources to initiate a proactive healing response involving your Immune System.

Principle of Advanced Natural Medicine #5:

Stress leads to Acidic Cellular Environments; Acidic Cellular Environments lead to damage; and damage always leads to the formation of Scar Tissue.

Principle of Advanced Natural Medicine #6:

When the amount of stress in our bodies and in our lives exceeds our Mitochondrial ability to produce energy, fatigue can be the only possible outcome.

Principle of Advanced Natural Medicine #7:

Energy will always go first where it is needed most. Your body—in its divine intelligence—has the ability to prioritize between immediately essential and secondarily essential functions.

Principle of Advanced Natural Medicine #8:

Let Organic food be thy medicine, and thy medicine be Organic food. Organic food tastes better because it is better.

—**Hippocrates** (Updated with a Modern Feel)

Principle of Advanced Natural Medicine #9:

More is not better—Better is better.

Principle of Advanced Natural Medicine #10:

Botanical Medicines reach their peak effectiveness when Mitochondria have everything they require to produce energy.

Principle of Advanced Natural Medicine #11:

The pH of a food is determined by what effect it has on pH inside of the body, not by its pH outside the body. Enzymes, nutrients, antioxidants, and the energy of the food will have a direct influence on the pH of the body, and can be reasonably measured using urinary and salivary pH testing methods.

Principle of Advanced Natural Medicine #12:

The better the flavor of a food, the more nutrients and *Chi* it possesses.

Principle of Advanced Natural Medicine #13:

Eat Something Green Every Day.

Principle of Advanced Natural Medicine #14:

Antioxidants stop damage before it starts.

Principle of Advanced Natural Medicine #15:

If it walks like a duck and talks like a duck… it's a duck.

Principle of Advanced Natural Medicine #16:

The number of poops per day should equal the number of major meals eaten per day. One poop per meal—that's the minimum.

Principle of Advanced Natural Medicine #17:

If it's not Organic, it's not food.

Principle of Advanced Natural Medicine #18:

Burn every calorie you consume every day.

Principle of Advanced Natural Medicine #19:

An adult body needs only one major meal each day to thrive energetically.

Principle of Advanced Natural Medicine #20:

Health is our ability to maximize the unification of our genetic potential with the energetic potential of our spirit, so as to achieve the personal development necessary to realize our dreams in this lifetime.

Principle of Advanced Natural Medicine #21:

When you do something positive for an organ the improved biochemical cellular functioning of that organ will often result in energy-cultivating emotional responses.

Principle of Advanced Natural Medicine #22:

Anything that leads to satisfaction cultivates healing energy.

Principle of Advanced Natural Medicine #23:

Love pain is a measurement of how much we really loved. The more it hurts, the more we loved—and that says something very special about us.

Principle of Advanced Natural Medicine #24:

Make life as easy as possible—Think Simple.

Principle of Advanced Natural Medicine #25:

Your body does not know how to lie—in your body lives only the truth.

Principle of Advanced Natural Medicine #26:

Belief is as essential to a Healing Process as any natural medicine.

Principle of Advanced Natural Medicine #27:

The only emotion that will ever come out of someone is what's already living within.

Principle of Advanced Natural Medicine #28:

The body is the densest form of energy, and as such, is the last place where degenerative disease will typically show itself. Degenerative disease can be traced back to its beginning, the disrupted flow of energy, and the Energy-Draining Reactions that result.

Principle of Advanced Natural Medicine #29:

The single most important factor in healing plan development is achieving the Therapeutic Range for Mitochondrial Energy Production.

Are you interested in studying more about Advanced Natural Medicine with Dr. Henele?

Contact Us:

GenesisHealing.net
ContactUs@GenesisHealing.net
Facebook—Henele E'ale

Classes Currently Being Offered:

Dr. Henele's Genesis Holistic Nutrition Program

- Offered Through Southwest Institute of the Healing Arts (www.SWIHA.edu) and Beginning in 2012 through Genesis at www.GenesisHealing.net.
- Study from the comfort of your home or any favorite hotspot without disrupting your existing schedule.
- Each weekly class includes a beautiful PowerPoint® presentation complete with Audio Narration by Dr. Henele and direct one-on-one interaction with your teacher.
- No Tests! We believe in learning through experience and positive, constructive feedback. *This is the new standard in Online Education.*
- Each week you will learn nutrition by Listening, Reading, Eating, and Interacting with your classmates and your teachers.
- **Level 1 Foundations** – (12 Weeks) – Exciting Class where students learn firsthand the powerful taste and feel of Organics. Topics: Optimizing Digestion, Proteins, Carbs, Lipids, Delayed Food Allergies, Vitamins, Antioxidants, Water, Chlorophyll, Minerals, Herbs.
- **Stress Management Tools** – (4 Weeks) – Breathing Techniques to help stabilize your Parasympathetic Nervous System (Scheduled to be added in 2012).
- **Botanical Medicines** – (4 Weeks) – Everyday Herbal solutions for Everyday problems (Scheduled to be added in 2012).
- **Nutritional Therapies** – (4 Weeks) - Define Exactly What is 'Eating Healthy' from your body's perspective.

- **Foundations 2** – (12 Weeks) – Exciting Class where students learn firsthand how to design Eating Healthy meals for virtually any health situation. Learn how to turn food into medicine. Topics include: Energetics, Energy Production, How to Heal each individual organ using Food as Medicine, and more.

- **Women's Health** – (6 Weeks) – Eating Healthy for Endometriosis, Ovarian Cysts, Menopause, Pregnancy, Et All (Scheduled to be added in 2012).

- **Weight Management & Eating Disorders** – (6 Weeks) – Our country has an epidemic that you can do something about. Learn how to bring the body back into a healthy weight balance while you develop a great relationship with your food.

- **Optimizing Your Supplementation** – (6 Weeks) – Learn which supplements are essential for you, how to select the best products, and how to take the correct amount for the correct situation.

- **Colon Cleansing & Cellular Detoxification Strategies** – (6 Weeks) – Learn how to clean your entire digestive tract and detoxify your Liver by actually doing it. Includes 4 week group cleanse and journaling exercises to chart your healing process along the way (Scheduled to be added in 2012).

- **Nutrition for High Performance Athletics** – (6 Weeks) – Learn the nutrition and dosing strategies necessary to maximize the 3 aspects of Athletics 1. Priming, 2. Competition, 3. Recovery (Scheduled to be added in 2012 or 2013).

- **Nutrition for Cancer Therapies** – (6 Weeks) – Learn how to function as a Holistic Integrative Nutritionist. Includes discussions on Advances in Chemotherapy and Radiation techniques as well as the Nutrients and dosing schedules essential to support a patient through most arduous treatments (Scheduled to be added in 2012 or 2013).

Release Point Therapy Program and Seminars

- Scheduled to begin running again in 2012.

- Study with Dr. Henele and learn how to use your hand to heal!

- This program is NCBTMB Certified.

- **Intro to Parasympathetic Techniques & Neck & Shoulder Protocol** – The Parasympathetic 'Rest & Digest' Nervous System is the gateway successful healers use to consistently access and balance the body's meridian energy fields. There is a distinctive art to engaging the Parasympathetics throughout a bodywork session that greatly amplifies the healing potential of touch. RPT Parasympathetic Techniques teach students from all disciplines how to enhance their healing skills and offers an introductory Release Point Therapy Protocol, the 9th of 10 Level 1 Release Point Therapy Protocols, for effectively treating neck and shoulder pain syndromes. This course is a pre-requisite for entry into the Release Point Therapy Program taught by Dr. Henele.

- **Release Point Therapy 1: Leg Protocol & Emotional Charge Assessment**– When assessing the obstacles to healing a practitioner can consider the presence of scar tissue, tissue acidity, biomechanical misalignment, and internalized emotional charge as obstacles to healing. Learn how to assess for emotional charge, scar tissue, acidic pH, and misalignment within minutes by reading their client's body. Additionally, this class teaches students the 1st of 10 Level 1 Release Point Therapy Protocols used to facilitate structural integration by clearing scar tissue and emotional charge.

- **Release Point Therapy 2: Thigh Protocol & Hip Protocol** – Did you know that people who have difficult times making decisions often have tight IT Bands and that the secret to healing low back pain is releasing the hips? Release Point Therapy 2 offers students Level 1 RPT Protocols 2 & 3 of 10 for addressing muscular imbalances in the thighs and hips that often contribute to pain syndromes in the upper portions of the body. Additionally, students learn how to master their RPT hand & elbow techniques for maximal effect in what can be a difficult area to work.

- **Release Point Therapy 3: Abdominal Protocol & Low Back Protocol**– Learn how to effectively decompress the spinal column by releasing the vaunted Psoas muscle from both the front and back of the body. Additionally, learn how to release scar tissue from the digestive tract as well as synergistic muscles and uniting muscles that often contribute to tension in the Psoas. This course is a must for any student interested in treating pain syndromes or professional athletes. Included in this course are the 4th and 5th of 10 Level 1 Release Point Therapy Protocols.

- **Release Point Therapy 4: Spine Protocol & Rib Cage Protocol** – How exactly, does one let go? What does it mean to let go of something? This class allows us to begin exploring some of the more spiritual aspects of healing though touch. In this class students will learn how to create space for spinal decompression and for (re)opening the heart energies. Techniques in this class are designed to help client's feel lighter, as if their spine and rip cage are floating within their skin. If you think this sounds good, wait until you feel it. Included in this course are the 6th and 7th of 10 Level 1 Release Point Therapy Protocols.

- **Release Point Therapy 5: Arm & Wrist Protocol & Jaw Protocol** – Many clients you will encounter experience frequent headaches, jaw clenching, carpel tunnel syndrome, etc. This class was designed with them in mind. Did you know that in order to overcome TMJ syndrome practitioners must treat the Triple Heater meridian in the forearms and the Lateral Pterygoid muscles? Did you know that tension in these two areas inhibits the body's production of Melatonin, our sleep hormone? When we treat the body thoroughly, addressing every possible area of scar tissue, misalignment, and emotional charge something miraculous happens...people get undeniably better. This class completes the classroom requirements for Level 1 Release Point Therapy certification by the Release Point Therapy Association. Included in this course are the 8th and 10th of 10 Level 1 Release Point Therapy Protocols.

Level 1 Certification Requirements

- Complete All Coursework in Level 1 Release Point Therapy, 125 Hours, including 20 Hours of Sessions Given.
- Demonstrate competency in each of the 10 RPT Protocols during Clinical Evaluation.
- Demonstrate competency in Emotional Charge and Scar Tissue Assessment during Clinical Evaluation.

AT LEAST 4% OF ALL NET PROCEEDS FROM *THE GREATEST ENERGY ALWAYS PREVAILS* IS DONATED TO SPONSOR CHILDREN IN NEED THROUGH ONE OF MY FAVORITE CHARITIES, FEED THE CHILDREN.

THANK YOU IN ADVANCE FOR HELPING TO MAKE A DIFFERENCE IN A CHILD'S LIFE.

FOR MORE INFORMATION ON HOW TO JOIN US IN BEING THE GREATEST ENERGY IN A CHILD'S LIFE, PLEASE VISIT WWW.FEEDTHECHILDREN.ORG.

TOGETHER WE CAN CREATE THE WORLD WHERE NO CHILD HAS TO GO HUNGRY.

RECOMMENDATIONS, REFERENCES, CITATIONS, AND CREDITS

RECOMMENDED ANATOMY

1. Netter, Frank H. *Atlas of Human Anatomy*. Philadelphia, PA: Saunders/Elsevier, 1999 2nd Ed. Print.

RECOMMENDED PHYSIOLOGY

1. Tortora, Gerard J. *Principles of Anatomy and Physiology*. Hoboken, NJ: J. Wiley, 2006. Print.

RECOMMENDED BIOCHEMISTRY

1. Berg, Jeremy M., John L. Tymoczko, Lubert Stryer, and Lubert Stryer. *Biochemistry*. New York: W.H. Freeman, 2007. Print.

2. Champe, Pamela C., Richard A. Harvey, and Denise R. Ferrier. *Biochemistry*. Philadelphia: Wolters Kluwer Health/Lippincott Williams & Wilkins, 2008. Print.

3. Evans, Joseph L. *The Secret Life of Mitochondria*. Xymogen. Print.

RECOMMENDED TRADITIONAL CHINESE MEDICINE

1. Beinfield, Harriet, and Efrem Korngold. Between Heaven and Earth: a Guide to Chinese Medicine. New York: Ballantine, 1991. Print.

2. Maciocia, Giovanni. Tongue Diagnosis in Chinese Medicine. Seattle: Eastland, 1995. Print.

RECOMMENDED NUTRITION

1. Emoto, Masaru. *The Secret Life of Water*. New York: Atria, 2005. Print.

2. Mateljan, George. *The World's Healthiest Foods: Essential Guide for the Healthiest Way of Eating*. Seattle, WA: George Mateljan Foundation, 2007. Print.

3. Pitchford, Paul. *Healing with Whole Foods: Oriental Traditions and Modern Nutrition*. Berkeley: North Atlantic Books, 1993. Print.

RECOMMENDED YOGA

1. Forrest, Ana T. *Fierce Medicine: Breakthrough Practices To Heal The Body And Ignite The Spirit*. New York: HarperCollins, 2011. Print.

2. Hirschi, Gertrud. Mudras: *Yoga In Your Hands*. Maine, Samuel Weiser, 2000. Print.

3. Iyengar, B.K.S. *Light on Pranayama: The Yogic Art of Breathing*. New York: Crossroad Publishing, 2005. Print.

4. Jois, Sri K. Pattabhi and Miele, Lino. *Astanga Yoga*. Italy: Miele, 2005. Print.

5. Muktibodhananda, Swami. *Hatha Yoga Pradipika*. India: Yoga Publications Trust, 2006. Print.

RECOMMENDED NATURAL HEALING

1. Angelou, Maya. *I Know Why The Caged Bird Sings*. New York: Bantam. 1969. Print.

2. Coelho, Paulo. *The Alchemist*. [San Francisco]: Harper: San Francisco, 1993. Print.

3. Desikachar, T. K. V., and Richard H. Cravens. *Health, Healing and Beyond: Yoga and the Living Tradition of Krishnamacharya*. New York: Aperture, 1998. Print.

4. Hahnemann, Samuel, B. K. Sarkar, and R. E. Dudgeon. *Organon of Medicine*. Delhi: Birla Publications, 2006. Print.

5. Jensen, DC, PhD, Bernard. *Iridology The Science and Practice in the Healing Arts. Vol. II*. Bernard Jensen. Print.

6. Lin, Derek. *The Tao of Daily Life & The Tao of Success*. New York: Penguin, 2007. Print.

7. Lindlahr, Henry. *Philosophy of Natural Therapeutics*. [Whitefish, Mont.?]: Kessinger Pub., [2000]. Print.

8. Parker, Ed. *Infinite Insights into Kenpo Volumes 1-5*. Los Angeles, Delsby, 1985. Print.

9. Pizzorno, Joseph E., and Michael T. Murray. *Textbook of Natural Medicine*. St. Louis, MO: Churchill Livingstone Elsevier, 2006. Print.

10. Rolf, Ida P., and Rosemary Feitis. *Ida Rolf Talks about Rolfing and Physical Reality*. New York: Harper & Row, 1978. Print.

11. Satchidananda, Sri Swami. *The Yoga Sutras of Patanjali*. Virginia: Integral Yoga Publications, 2005. Print.

12. Seuss, Dr. *Oh, The Places You Will Go!* and *It's A Great Day For UP!* New York: Random House, 1971. Print.

13. Tsunetomo, Yamamoto and Wilson, William Scott. Hagakure: *The Book of the Samurai. Japan: Kodansha America, 1979*. Print.

REFERENCES

1. Abeloff, Martin D. *Clinical Oncology*. Philadelphia, PA: Elsevier Churchill Livingstone, 2004. Print.

2. Adamo, Peter. *Eat Right for Your Type*. New York: BG.P. Putnam's Sons, 1996. Print.

3. Alschuler, Lise, Karolyn A. Gazella, and Lise Alschuler. *The Definitive Guide to Cancer: an Integrative Approach to Prevention, Treatment, and Healing*. New York: Celestial Arts, 2010. Print.

4. Anderson, Richard. *Cleanse & Purify Thyself*. Books 1 & 2 Medford, Or.: Christobe Pub., 2007. Print.

5. Anderson, ND, NMD, Rich. *The Liver*. Mt. Shasta, CA: Christobe, 1999. Print.

6. Appleton, Nancy. *Lick the Sugar Habit.* Garden City Park, NY: Avery Pub. Group, 1996. Print.

7. Begley, Ed. *Living like Ed.* New York: Clarkson Potter, 2008. Print.

8. Bernstein, Richard K. *Dr. Bernstein's Diabetes Solution: the Complete Guide to Achieving Normal Blood Sugars.* New York: Little, Brown and, 2007. Print.

9. Bernstein, Richard K. *The Diabetes Diet: Dr. Bernstein's Low-carbohydrate Solution.* New York: Little, Brown and, 2005. Print.

10. Boyle, Wade, and André Saine. *Lectures in Naturopathic Hydrotherapy.* East Palestine, OH: Buckeye Naturopathic, 1988. Print.

11. Breiner, Mark A. *Whole-body Dentistry: Discover the Missing Piece to Better Health.* Fairfield, CT: Quantum Health, 1999. Print.

12. Brennan, Barbara Ann. *Hands of Light: a Guide to Healing through the Human Energy Field.* Toronto: Bantam, 1988. Print.

13. Bruyere, Rosalyn L. *Wheels of Light: Chakras, Auras, and the Healing Energy of the Body.* New York: Fireside Book, 1994. Print.

14. Cabot, Sandra. *The Liver Cleansing Diet.* Glendale, AZ: S.C.B. International, 2008. Print.

15. Chevallier, Andrew. *Natural Health Encyclopedia of Herbal Medicine.* New York: DK Pub., 2000. Print.

16. Chia, Mantak. *Chi Nei Tsang: Internal Organ Chi Massage.* Huntington, NY: Healing Tao, 1990. Print.

17. Cichoke, DC, Anthony. Bromelain. *New Canaan, CT: Keats,* 1998. Print.

18. Dadd-Redalia, Debra. *Home Safe Home: Protecting Yourself and Your Family from Everyday Toxics and Harmful Household Products.* New York: Jeremy P. Tarcher/Putnams, 1997. Print.

19. Desikachar, T. K. V. *The Heart of Yoga: Developing a Personal Practice.* Rochester, VT: Inner Traditions International, 1999. Print.

20. Dorfman, Kelly. *What's Eating Your Child?: the Hidden Connections between Food and Childhood Ailments : Anxiety, Recurrent Ear Infections, Stomachaches, Picky Eating, Rashes, ADHD, and More : and What Every Parent Can Do about It.* New York, NY: Workman Pub., 2011. Print.

21. Dougans, Inge. *The Complete Illustrated Guide to Reflexology: Therapeutic Foot Massage for Health and Well-being.* Shaftesbury, Dorset: Element, 1996. Print.

22. Dychtwald, Ken. *Bodymind.* New York: Pantheon, 1977. Print.

23. Elkins, Rita. *Bilberry*. Pleasent Grove, UT: Woodland, 1998. Print.

24. Elkins, Rita. *Chinese Red Yeast Rice*. Pleasent Grove, UT: Woodland, 1998. Print.

25. Elkins, Rita. *Hawaiian Noni*. Pleasant Grove, UT: Woodland, 1998. Print.

26. Emoto, Masaru. *The Hidden Messages in Water*. Hillsboro, Or.: Beyond Words Pub., 2004. Print.

27. Frawley, David. *Ayurveda and the Mind: the Healing of Consciousness*. Twin Lakes, WI: Lotus, 1997. Print.

28. Gerson, Charlotte; Walker, Morton. *The Gerson Therapy: The Proven Nutritional Program For Cancer and Other Illnesses*. New York: Kensington, 2006. Print.

29. Gerson, Max. *A Cancer Therapy: Results of Fifty Cases*. Bonita, CA: Gerson Institute, 1986. Print.

30. Gilbert, Kate. *Cordyceps Sinensis*. Pleasant Grove, Utah: Woodland, 2000. Print.

31. Gittleman, Ann Louise. *Guess What Came to Dinner?: Parasites and Your Health*. New York: Avery, 2001. Print.

32. Gore, Albert. *An Inconvenient Truth: the Planetary Emergency of Global Warming and What We Can Do about It*. New York: Rodale, 2006. Print.

33. Gottschall, Elaine Gloria. *Breaking the Vicious Cycle: Intestinal Health through Diet*. Baltimore, Ont.: Kirkton, 2007. Print.

34. Grandgeorge, Didier. *The Spirit of Homeopathic Medicines: Essential Insights to 300 Remedies*. Berkeley, CA: North Atlantic, 1998. Print.

35. Green, James. *The Herbal Medicine-makers' Handbook: a Home Manual*. Freedom, CA: Crossing, 2000. Print.

36. Hansen, John T., Bruce M. Koeppen, and Frank H. Netter. *Netter's Atlas of Human Physiology*. Teterboro, NJ: Icon Learning Systems, 2002. Print.

37. Hay, Louise L. *You Can Heal Your Life*. Santa Monica, CA: Hay House, 1987. Print.

38. Hass, Elson M. *Staying Healthy with Nutrition*. Berkeley: Celestial, 2006. Print.

39. Hesse, Hermann, and Hilda Rosner. *Siddhartha*. Toronto: Bantam, 1971. Print.

40. Hobbs, L.Ac., Christopher. *Medical Mushrooms*. Summertown, Tennessee: Botanica, 1986. Print.

41. Holmes, Peter. *The Energetics of Western Herbs: Treatment Strategies Integrating Western and Oriental Herbal Medicine*. Boulder, CO: Snow Lotus, 2006. Print.

42. Howell, Edward, and Maynard Murray. *Enzyme Nutrition: the Food Enzyme Concept*. Wayne, NJ: Avery Pub. Group, 1985. Print.

43. Hudson, Tori. *Women's Encyclopedia of Natural Medicine: Alternative Therapies and Integrative Medicine for Total Health and Wellness.* New York: McGraw-Hill, 2008. Print.

44. Huggins, Hal A. *It's All in Your Head: the Link between Mercury Amalgams and Illness.* Garden City Park, NY: Avery Pub. Group, 1993. Print.

45. Inkeles, Gordon, and Murray Todris. *The Art of Sensual Massage.* New York: Simon and Schuster, 1972. Print.

46. Iyengar, B.K.S. *Light on Yoga: Yoga Dipika.* New York: Schocken, 1979. Print.

47. Jensen, DC, PhD, Bernard. *Dr Jensen's Guide to Better Bowel Care.* Bernard Jensen. Print.

48. Jensen, Bernard. *Dr. Jensen's Guide to Body Chemistry & Nutrition.* Los Angeles: Keats Pub., 2000. Print.

49. Kent, J. T. *Lectures on Homeopathic Philosophy.* Berkeley, CA: North Atlantic, 1979. Print.

50. Kilham, Chris. *OPC: The Miracle Antioxidant.* Los Angeles: Keats, 1997. Print.

51. Kushi, Michio, Aveline Kushi, and Alex Jack. *Macrobiotic Diet.* Tokyo: Japan Publications, 1993. Print.

52. Kushi, Michio, William Tara, David Lasocki, and David Elliott. *Your Face Never Lies.* Wayne, NJ: Avery Group, 1983. Print.

53. Lad, Vasant. *Ayurveda: the Science of Self Healing.* Twin Lakes, WI: Lotus, 2009. Print.

54. Lark, MD, Susan M. *Natural Treatment of Fibroid Tumors and Endometriosis.* New Canaan, CT: Keats, 1996. Print.

55. Lee, John R., and Virginia Hopkins. *What Your Doctor May Not Tell You about Menopause: the Breakthrough Book on Natural Progesterone.* New York, NY: Warner, 1996. Print.

56. Lee, Richard. *Pocket Manual of Chinese Medicine.* Woodland Hills, CA (4491 Deanwood Dr, CA 91364): Lucky Dog Pub., 1998. Print.

57. Lee, PhD, Willian. *Coenzyme Q-10.* New Canaan, CT: Keats, 1987. Print.

58. Ley, PhD, Beth M. *Castor Oil!* Detroit Lakes: BL Publications, 2003. Print.

59. Lidell, Lucy, Narayani Rabinovitch, and Giris Rabinovitch. *The Sivananda Companion to Yoga.* New York: Simon and Schuster, 1983. Print.

60. Majeed, PhD, Muhammed. *Tumeric and the Healing Cucruminoids.* New Canaan, CT: Keats, 1996. Print.

61. Marz, R. *Medical Nutrition from Marz.* [S.l.]: Omnivite Nutrition, 1999. Print.

62. McGarey, Analea. *Born to Heal: the Life Story of Holistic Pioneer Gladys Taylor McGarey, M.D.* Scottsdale, AZ: Inkwell Productions, 2003. Print.

63. Meyerowitz, Steve, and F. Batmanghelidj. *Water: the Ultimate Cure.* Summertown, TN: Distributed Book Pub., 2000. Print.

64. Meyerowitz, Steve. *Wheatgrass, Nature's Finest Medicine: the Complete Guide to Using Grass, Foods & Juices to Help Your Health.* Great Barrington, MA: Sproutman Publications, 1999. Print.

65. Milne, Robert D., Blake More, and Burton Goldberg. *Definitive Guide to Headaches: an Alternative Medicine.* Tiburon, CA: Future Medicine Pub., 1997. Print.

66. Mindell, PhD, Earl. Garlic: *The Miracle Nutrient.* New Canaan, CT: Keats, 1996. Print.

67. Moore, Keith L., Marlene Herbst, and Megan Thompson. *Essentials of Human Embryology.* Toronto: B.C. Decker, 1988. Print.

68. Moss, Ralph W., and Ralph W. Moss. *The Cancer Industry: the Classic Expose on the Cancer Establishment.* New York: Paragon House, 1991. Print.

69. Murray, Michael T., Joseph E. Pizzorno, and Lara Pizzorno. *The Encyclopedia of Healing Foods.* New York: Atria, 2005. Print.

70. Murray, Michael T. *The Encyclopedia of Nutritional Supplements.* New York: Three Rivers Press, 1996. Print.

71. Myss, Caroline M. *Anatomy of the Spirit: the Seven Stages of Power and Healing.* New York: Harmony, 1996. Print.

72. Norten, Ellen, and Jean Pütz. *Neem: India's Miraculous Healing Plant.* Rochester, VT: Healing Arts, 2000. Print.

73. Ostrander, Sheila, Lynn Schroeder, and Nancy Ostrander. *Super Learning.* New York: Delacorte, 1979. Print.

74. Painter, Jack W. *Deep Bodywork and Personal Development.* Mill Valley: Bodymind, 1989. Print.

75. Parham, Peter. *The Immune System.* New York: Garland Publishing, 2000. Print.

76. Perlmutter, David. *The Better Brain Book.* New York: Riverhead Books, 2005. Print.

77. Preuss, Harry G., and Sensuke Konno. *Maitake Magic: Maitake Mushroom Fractions: Capture the Force of Nature's Amazing Powerful Immune Boosters, Cancer Protectors, and Metabolic Activators.* Topanga, CA: Freedom, 2002. Print.

78. Rama, Swami, Rudolph Ballentine, M.D., and Alan Hymes, M.D. *Science of Breath.* Honesdale, Pennsylvania: Himalayan Institute, 1998. Print.

79. Rector-Page, Linda, N.D., *Healthy Healing.* USA: Healthy Healing pub, 1992. Print.

80. Rolf, Ida P. *Rolfing: Reestablishing the Natural Alignment and Structural Integration of the Human Body for Vitality and Well-being.* Rochester, VT: Healing Arts, 1989. Print.

81. Robbins, Stanley L., Ramzi S. Cotran, and Vinay Kumar. *Pathology Basis of Disease.* Philadelphia: W.B. Saunders, 1989. Print.

82. Roberts, Susan M. *Naturopathic Pediatric Essentials.* Wenatchee, WA: Healing Mountain Pub., 2003. Print.

83. Ross, Julia. *The Mood Cure: the 4-step Program to Rebalance Your Emotional Chemistry and Rediscover Your Natural Sense of Well-being.* New York: Viking, 2002. Print.

84. Sankey, Mikio. *Esoteric Acupuncture.* Inglewood, CA: Mountain Castle Pub., 2002. Print.

85. Schulze, Richard. *25 Ways to Have the Cleanest Liver: Dr. Schulze Answers Your Questions about Liver Cleansing.* Marina Del Rey, CA: Natural Healing Publications, 2004. Print.

86. Schulze, Richard. *Breaking the Code: a Layperson's Guide to Unlocking the Secret World of Medical Terminology.* Santa Monica, CA: Natural Healing Publications, 2001. Print.

87. Schulze, Richard. *Common Sense Health and Healing: 20 Simple, Easy and Powerful Steps to Create a New Healthy Life.* Santa Monica, CA: Natural Healing Publications, 2002. Print.

88. Schulze, Richard. *There Are No Incurable Diseases: Dr. Richard Schulze's 30-day Intensive Cleansing and Detoxification Program.* Santa Monica, CA: Natural Healing Publications, 1999. Print.

89. Schlosser, Eric. *Fast Food Nation: the Dark Side of the All-American Meal.* Boston: Houghton Mifflin, 2001. Print.

90. Selye, Hans. *The Stress of Life.* New York: McGraw-Hill, 1956. Print.

91. Simpson, Liz. *The Book of Crystal Healing.* New York: Sterling Pub., 1997. Print.

92. Skousen, Max B. *Aloe Vera.* Cameron Park, CA: Aloe Vera Research Institute, 1992. Print.

93. Steinmand, David, and Michael Wisner. *Living Healthy in a Toxic World.* USA: Time Warner International, 1997. Print.

94. Sylver, PhD, Nina. *The Holistic Handbook of Sauna Therapy*. Stone Ridge, NY: Center for Frequency Education, 2004. Print.

95. Trenev, Natasha. *Probiotics: Nature's Internal Healers*. Garden City Park, NY: Avery Pub. Group, 1998. Print.

96. Upledger, John E., and Jon D. Vredevoogd. *Craniosacral Therapy*. Seattle: Eastland, 2002. Print.

97. Vithoulkas, George. *The Science of Homeopathy*. New York: Grove, 1980. Print.

98. Wallach, Joel D., and Ma Lan. *Rare Earths: Forbidden Cures*. Bonita, CA: Double Happiness Pub., 1994. Print.

99. Walsch, Neale Donald. *Conversations with God: an Uncommon Dialogue: Book 2*. Norfolk, VA: Hampton Roads, 1997. Print.

100. Werbach, Melvyn R. *Healing through Nutrition: a Natural Approach to Treating 50 Common Illnesses with Diet and Nutrients*. New York, NY: HarperCollins, 1993. Print.

101. Winter, Ruth. *A Consumer's Dictionary of Cosmetic Ingredients: Complete Information about the Harmful and Desirable Ingredients Found in Cosmetics and Cosmeceuticals*. New York: Three Rivers, 2009. Print.

102. Winter, Ruth. *A Consumer's Dictionary of Food Additives*. New York: Three Rivers, 2009. Print.

103. Wolcott, William L., and Trish Fahey. *The Metabolic Typing Diet*. New York: Doubleday, 2000. Print.

104. Ziff, Sam, and Michael F. Ziff. *Dentistry without Mercury*. Orlando, FL: Bio-Probe, 2001. Print.

105. Ziff, Sam, Michael F. Ziff, and Mats Hanson. *Dental Mercury Detox*. Orlando, FL: Bio-Probe, 2001. Print.

CITATIONS

Biochem J. 1996 January 1; 313(Pt 1): 207–213.
Oxygen and pH regulation of protein synthesis in mitochondria from Artemia franciscana embryos.
K E Kwast and S C Hand
Department of Environmental, Population, and Organismic Biology, University of Colorado, Boulder 80309-0334, USA.

Mitochondiral Function as a Target for Alzhemier's Disease
Organizers: Howard Fillit (Alzheimer's Drug Discovery Foundation) and Sonya Dougal (The New York Academy of Sciences)Presented by the Alzheimer's Drug Discovery Foundation, the Brain Dysfunction Discussion Group, and The New York Academy of Sciences.
Reported by Catherine Zandonella | Posted July 6, 2010

Saturated but not mono-unsaturated fatty acids induce apoptotic cell death in neonatal rat ventricular myocytes JE de Vries, MM Vork, TH Roemen, YF de Jong, JP Cleutjens, GJ van der Vusse and M van Bilsen Department of Physiology, Cardiovascular Research Institute Maastricht , Maastricht University, The Netherlands.

Methylmercury-induced changes in Mitochondrial function in striatal synaptosomes are calcium-dependent and ros-independent
Anne Dreiem[1*] and Richard F. Seegal[1,2]
[1]New York State Department of Health, Wadsworth Center, Albany, NY
[2]School of Public Health, University at Albany, Albany, NY
[*]Present address: Institut Curie-Recherche, Bâts. 110–112, Centre Universitaire U-612 INSERM, Génotoxicologie, Signalisation et Radiothérapie Expérimentale 91405 Orsay Cedex (France)
Corresponding author: Richard F. Seegal New York State Department of Health Wadsworth Center, Empire State Plaza Albany, NY 12201 Phone: 518 474 7279 Fax: 518 486 1505 E-mail: seegal@wadsworth.org

1. Trifunovic A, Wredenberg A, Falkenberg M, Spelbrink J N, Rovio A T, Bruder C E, Bohlooly-Y M, Gidlöf S, Oldfors A, Wibom R, Törnell J, Jacobs HT, Larsson N G. Premature ageing in mice expressing defective mitochondrial DNA polymerase. Nature 429(6990): 417-423, 2004.

2. Falkenberg M, Gaspari M, Rantanen A, Trifunovic A, Larsson NG, Gustafsson CM. Mitochondrial transcription factors B1 and B2 activate transcription of human mtDNA. Nat Genet. 13(9): 935-944, 2004.

3. Balzarini J, Pérez-Pérez M, San-Félix A, Velázquez S, Camarasa M, Perno C, De Clerq E, Anderson J, Karlsson A. Exploitation of the low fidelity of HIV-1 reverse tran-scriptase and the nucleotide composition bias in the HIV-1 genome to alter the drug-resistance spectrum of HIV. J. Virol. 75: 5772-5777, 2001.

(*American Journal of Pathology*. 2010;177:447-455.)
© 2010 American Society for Investigative Pathology
DOI: 10.2353/ajpath.2010.091029 High Glucose Disrupts Mitochondrial Morphology in Retinal Endothelial Cells Implications for Diabetic Retinopathy
Kyle Trudeau*, Anthony J.A. Molina*, Wen Guo* and Sayon Roy* From the Departments of Medicine,* and Ophthalmology, Boston University School of Medicine, Massachusetts

Tetrahydrocannabinol disrupts mitochondrial function and cell energetics
Theodore A. Sarafian, Shaghig Kouyoumjian, Farnaz Khoshaghideh, Donald P. Tashkin, and Michael D. Roth
Department of Medicine, Division of Pulmonary and Critical Care, Center for Health Sciences, University of California, Los Angeles, Los Angeles, California 90095
Submitted 20 May 2002; accepted in final form 11 October 2002 *Am J Physiol Lung Cell Mol Physiol* 284: L298–L306, 2003.
First published October 25, 2002; 10.1152/ajplung.00157.2002.

Disruption of Mitochondrial Function and Cellular ATP Levels by Amiodarone and *N*-Desethylamiodarone in Initiation of Amiodarone-Induced Pulmonary Cytotoxicity
M. W. Bolt1, J. W. Card1, W. J. Racz1, J. F. Brien1 and T. E. Massey[1,2,3]
Author Affiliations- Departments of [1]Pharmacology and Toxicology (M.W.B., J.W.C., W.J.R., J.F.B., T.E.M.) and [2]Medicine (T.E.M.), and [3]School of Environmental Studies (T.E.M.), Queen's University, Kingston, Ontario, Canada
Dr. Thomas E. Massey, Department of Pharmacology and Toxicology, Botterell Hall Room 535, Queen's University, Kingston, ON, Canada, K7L 3N6.
E-mail:masseyt@post.queensu.ca

Disruption of Mitochondrial Function by Suramin Measured by Rhodamine 123 Retention and Oxygen Consumption in Intact DUI45 Prostate Carcinoma Cells I
Randall P. Rago, Peter C. Brazy, and George Wiiding 2
William S. Middleton Veteran's Hospital [R. P. R., P. C. B., G. W.], University of Wisconsin Comprehensive Cancer Center [R. P. R., G. W.], and Department ofMedicine [P. C. B.], University of Wisconsin Hospitals and Clinics, Madison, Wisconsin 53792

Effects of cortisol on the levels of metabolites and enzymes controlling glucose production from pyruvateW. Seubert[a], H.V. Henning[a], W. Schoner[a] and M. L'age[a] Institut für vegetative Physiologie, Chemisch-physiologisches Institut der Universität, Frankfurt/Main, Germany Available online 12 November 2002. J Cell Physiol. 1988 Sep;136(3):507-13.

REFERENCED WEBSITES OF INTEREST

1. World's Healthiest Foods - http://whfoods.org/
2. Nutrition Data - http://nutritiondata.self.com/
3. Linus Pauling Institute - http://lpi.oregonstate.edu/
4. Environmental Working Group – http://www.ewg.org/
5. National Resource Defense Council – http://www.nrdc.org
6. Sierra Club - http://www.sierraclub.org/
7. National Geographic - http://www.nationalgeographic.com/
8. ORAC Watch - http://www.oracwatch.org/
9. ORAC Values - http://www.oracvalues.com/
10. GoodFood World - http://www.goodfoodworld.com/2010/12/top-organic-food-and-farming-trends-in-2011/
11. World Life Expectancy - http://www.worldlifeexpectancy.com/
12. Mitochondrial Cell Respiration - http://biology.clc.uc.edu/Courses/bio104/cellresp.htm
13. Obesity Society - http://www.obesity.org/
14. Neuroscience Made Easy - http://faculty.washington.edu/chudler/what.html
15. The Literacy Company - http://www.readfaster.com/education_stats.asp
16. Wikipedia
17. YouTube

PHOTO CREDITS

1. Cover Photo Credit Alexia Bauer

2. Cover Models: Dr. Henele, Ashley Bush

3. Chapter 6 Meridian Illustrations - Jaclyn Bain

4. The License For All Photo Used Within This Text Have Either Been Purchased Royalty-Free From ThinkStock.com or ShutterStock.com or granted permission for use through agreements established between the creator and WikiCommons.org.

5. All Tables, Graphs and Meridian Illustrations from Chapter 6 are the intellectual property of Dr. Henele and Genesis Health Systems, PLLC.

Figure 1.1 – ThinkStock.com – Hemera
Figure 2.1 – Genesis Health Systems – Dr. Henele
Figure 2.2 – Genesis Health Systems – Dr. Henele
Figure 3.2 – Genesis Health Systems – Dr. Henele
Figure 3.2 – ShutterStock.com – Alila Sao Mai
Figure 3.3 – ShutterStock.com
Figure 3.4 – ShutterStock.com
Figure 3.5 – Genesis Health Systems – Dr. Henele
Figure 3.7 – Genesis Health Systems – Dr. Henele
Figure 3.8 – ShutterStock.com
Figure 3.9 – Genesis Health Systems – Dr. Henele
Figure 3.10 – ShutterStock.com
Figure 4.1 – ThinkStock.com – Michal Sz
Figure 4.2 – ShutterStock.com
Figure 4.3 – ThinkStock.com – Michal Sz
Figure 4.4 – WikiCommons.org
Figure 4.5 – WikiCommons.org
Figure 4.6A – WikiCommons.org
Figure 4.6B – WikiCommons.org
Figure 5.1 – Courtesy of USGOVERNMENTSPENDING.ORG
Figure 5.2 - ShutterStock.com – Alila Sao Mai
Figure 5.3 - ShutterStock.com – Blamb
Figure 5.4 – Genesis Health Systems – Dr. Henele
Figure 5.5 – Genesis Health Systems – Dr. Henele
Figure 5.6 – Genesis Health Systems – Dr. Henele
Figure 5.7 – Genesis Health Systems – Dr. Henele
Figure 6.1 – Genesis Health Systems – Dr. Henele
Figure 6.2 – Genesis Health Systems – Dr. Henele
Figure 6.3 – Genesis Health Systems – Dr. Henele

SPECIAL THANKS FOR THE HEALING SOUNDS & LAUGHTER

My Healing Work Isn't Possible Without Your Wisdom – Dr. H.

Bob Marley
Richard Pryor
Miles Davis
Michael Jackson
Marvin Gaye
Quincy Jones
Stevie Wonder
Santana
Jamiroquai
Sade
Eddie Murphy
Samantha James
Ryan Leslie
Alicia Keys
Vikter Duplaix
Erykah Badu
Bebel Gilberto
Jill Scott
Kanye West
4 Hero
Blue Six
Diana Krall
Musiq
Zero 7
Israel Kamakawiwo'ole
Keali'I Reichel
Kirk Franklin
Luther Vandross
Isley Brothers
Julian 'Cannonball' Adderley – ***74 Miles Away, Best Jazz Recording of All-Time!***

INDEX